# Register Now for Online Access to Your Book

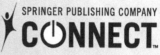

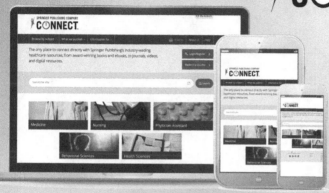

Your print purchase of *Empowerment Strategies for Nurses, Second Edition* **includes online access to the contents of your book**—increasing accessibility, portability, and searchability!

## Access today at:

http://connect.springerpub.com/content/book/978-0-8261-6792-7
**or scan the QR code at the right with your smartphone and enter the access code below.**

**4RCXAHGU**

*Scan here for quick access.*

# Empowerment Strategies for Nurses

**Margaret McAllister, EdD, RN,** is professor of nursing at Central Queensland University, Australia. A fellow of the Australian College of Mental Health Nursing and of the College of Nursing, Australia, she is widely published internationally in nursing. With a long background in mental health nursing, Dr. McAllister became conscious of the importance of empathy, acceptance, optimism, and compassionate action early in her career and has continued to teach and develop these concepts for nurses directly in classroom and online teaching as well as in research. Her 2009 paper on teaching and learning resilience continues to be highly cited. In 2010, Dr. McAllister was honored with an Australian Learning and Teaching Council Citation for the development of the practical theoretical concept, Solution Focused Nursing, as an effective way of developing high-level caring skills in nurses. As well as teaching within a Master of Mental Health Nursing program, Dr. McAllister leads a vibrant research network on Narratives of Health and Wellbeing at Central Queensland University and is a strategic leader in the Arts Health Network, Queensland. She has coauthored several books: *The Clinical Helper, Stories in Mental Health*, and *Solution-Focused Nursing*. She has published over 150 refereed journal articles and her work has been cited by others more than 2,000 times. She has supervised diverse nursing research projects, including nursing history, stress and shame in nursing, narratives of practice, and innovative arts-based interventions for empathy and well-being.

**Donna Lee Brien, PhD,** is professor of creative industries at Central Queensland University, Australia. She is an award-winning educator in creative writing and publishing. A member of the multidisciplinary research group on Narratives of Health and Wellbeing at Central Queensland University, she has authored over 20 books and exhibition catalogues and has published over 200 journal articles and scholarly book chapters. Dr. Brien is also a highly experienced editor and is currently the coeditor of *The Australasian Journal of Popular Culture*. Her most recent books are *Recovering History Through Fact and Fiction: Forgotten Lives* (with Dallas John Baker and Nike Sulway), *Offshoot: Contemporary Life Writing Methodologies and Practice* (with Quinn Eades), and *The Routledge Companion to Literature and Food* (with Lorna Piatti-Farnell). Dr. Brien has been collaborating with Professor Margaret McAllister on interdisciplinary research projects in the Health Humanities and Arts and Health areas since 2012.

# Empowerment Strategies for Nurses

## Developing Resilience in Practice

## Second Edition

*Margaret McAllister, EdD, RN*

*Donna Lee Brien, PhD*

**Editors**

**SPRINGER PUBLISHING COMPANY**

Springer Publishing Company, LLC
11 West 42nd Street
New York, NY 10036
www.springerpub.com
http://connect.springerpub.com

*Acquisitions Editor*: Joe Morita
*Compositor*: Exeter Premedia Services Private Ltd.

*ISBN*: 978-0-8261-6789-7
*ebook ISBN*: 978-0-8261-6792-7
*Instructor's Manual ISBN*: 978-0-8261-6447-6
*Instructor's PowerPoints ISBN*: 978-0-8261-6449-0
*DOI*: 10.1891/9780826167927

*Instructor's Materials: Qualified instructors may request supplements by emailing textbook@springerpub.com*

19 20 21 22 / 5 4 3 2 1

The author and the publisher of this Work have made every effort to use sources believed to be reliable to provide information that is accurate and compatible with the standards generally accepted at the time of publication. Because medical science is continually advancing, our knowledge base continues to expand. Therefore, as new information becomes available, changes in procedures become necessary. We recommend that the reader always consult current research and specific institutional policies before performing any clinical procedure. The author and publisher shall not be liable for any special, consequential, or exemplary damages resulting, in whole or in part, from the readers' use of, or reliance on, the information contained in this book. The publisher has no responsibility for the persistence or accuracy of URLs for external or third-party Internet websites referred to in this publication and does not guarantee that any content on such websites is, or will remain, accurate or appropriate.

**Library of Congress Cataloging-in-Publication Data**

Names: McAllister, Margaret, RN, editor. | Brien, Donna Lee, 1959- editor.
Title: Empowerment strategies for nurses: developing resilience in practice
    / Margaret McAllister, Donna Lee Brien, editors.
Other titles: Resilient nurse.
Description: Second edition. | New York, NY: Springer Publishing Company,
    [2020] | Preceded by Resilient nurse / Margaret McAllister, John B. Lowe,
    editors. c2011. | Includes bibliographical references and index.
Identifiers: LCCN 2019010259| ISBN 9780826167897 | ISBN 9780826167927
    (e-book) | ISBN 9780826164476 (instructors manual) | ISBN 9780826164490
    (instructors Powerpoints)
Subjects: | MESH: Nursing | Nurses—psychology | Vocational Guidance |
    Resilience, Psychological | Nurse's Role | Adaptation, Psychological
Classification: LCC RT82 | NLM WY 16.1 | DDC 610.73—dc23
LC record available at https://lccn.loc.gov/2019010259

Margaret McAllister: https://orcid.org/0000-0003-1181-1610
Donna Lee Brien: https://orcid.org/0000-0002-9005-3645

*To the many nurses who, in their efforts to support the
health and well-being of patients, confront challenges,
yet are able to persevere, thrive, and be
an inspiration to us all.*

# Contents

# Contributors

**Edward Aquin, RN, MN,** Lecturer in Nursing, School of Nursing, Australian Catholic University, Melbourne, Australia

**Jane Brannan, EdD, RN, CNE,** Professor of Nursing, WellStar School of Nursing, Kennesaw State University, Kennesaw, Georgia

**Donna Lee Brien, PhD,** Professor of Creative Industries, School of Education and the Arts, Central Queensland University Australia, Noosaville, Queensland, Australia

**Adam Burston, PhD, RN, MHSM,** Lecturer in Nursing, Australian Catholic University, Brisbane, Australia

**Sherry S. Chesak, PhD, RN,** Assistant Professor of Nursing, College of Medicine, Mayo Clinic, Rochester, Minnesota

**Mary de Chesnay, PhD, RN, PMHCNS-BC, FAAN,** Professor Emerita, WellStar School of Nursing, Kennesaw State University, Kennesaw, Georgia

**Susanne Cutshall, DNP, RN, CNS,** Assistant Professor of Medicine and Nursing, Mayo College of Medicine, Rochester, Minnesota

**Andrew Estefan, PhD, MN, BN, RPN, DipNSc,** Associate Professor, Psychiatric Nursing, Faculty of Nursing, University of Calgary, Calgary, Alberta, Canada

**Kim Foster, PhD, MA, BN, RN, DipAppSc,** Professor of Mental Health Nursing, School of Nursing, Midwifery and Paramedicine, Australian Catholic University, and NorthWestern Mental Health, Melbourne Health, Parkville, Victoria, Australia

**Ben Hannigan, PhD, RN,** Professor of Mental Health Nursing, School of Healthcare Sciences, Cardiff University, Cardiff, Wales, UK

**Julie Hanson, PhD, RN,** Lecturer in Nursing, School of Nursing, Midwifery and Paramedic Science, University of the Sunshine Coast, Maroochydore, Queensland, Australia

**Patricia L. Hart, RN, PhD,** Associate Professor of Nursing, Coordinator of the MSN Education program, Kennesaw State University, Kennesaw, Georgia

**Mary Katsikitis, PhD, BA (Hons),** Professor of Psychology, University of the Sunshine Coast, Maroochydore, Queensland, Australia

**Margaret McAllister, EdD, RN,** Professor of Nursing, School of Nursing, Midwifery and Social Sciences, Central Queensland University Australia, Noosaville, Queensland, Australia

**Katherine Pachkowski, PhD, RN,** Associate Professor in Psychiatric Nursing, Brandon University, Brandon, Manitoba, Canada

**Teddie Potter, PhD, RN, FAAN,** Clinical Professor, School of Nursing, University of Minnesota, Minneapolis, Minnesota

**Rachael R. Sharman, PhD,** Senior Lecturer in Psychology, University of the Sunshine Coast, Maroochydore, Australia

**Sandra Sharp, PhD, RN,** Senior Lecturer in Nursing, School of Health and Social Care, Napier University, Edinburgh, Scotland

**Linda Shields, PhD, MMedSci, BAppSci (Nursing), FCNA, FRSM,** Professor of Rural Health, Charles Sturt University, Bathurst, New South Wales, Australia

**Anthony Tuckett, PhD, RN,** Associate Professor, School of Nursing, Midwifery and Social Work, University of Queensland, Brisbane, Queensland, Australia

# Foreword

In the last decade, technology, social media, and globalization have had huge impacts on the way our community operates, on the way news is reported, and on the way we interact with others. Migration patterns, whereby millions of people around the world are being displaced from their countries of origin due to war, famine, and environmental disaster, are likely to continue into the future, and the developed nations will increasingly need to respond to these challenges. Uncertainty and rapid change will have an effect on the health and mental health needs of the community. In order to face the challenges ahead and flourish, we need to intentionally develop and cultivate the resilience of the population.

Nurses will be key to constructing and supporting more resilient communities, and this book, *Empowerment Strategies for Nurses: Developing Resilience in Practice*, Second Edition, is a valuable resource in nurses' efforts to do that. Importantly, and as a first step, nurses need to develop personal resilience and support those we work with to do the same. As supporters, carers, navigators, and interpreters of the healthcare system, nurses have a particularly important role within that system. While of course nurses work as part of a team, within that team individual nurses often take on many roles at the same time they provide people what they need, in the way that they want it, all within a too-busy workplace that has its own demands. As a result, nursing work can be stressful, overwhelming, and exhausting. How can a nurse provide person-centered care in a kind, caring, and compassionate way if his or her fuel tank is empty?

It is not an indulgence for nurses to look after themselves, to nurture themselves, in order that they can more effectively provide care to others—in fact, it is essential; that is why this book is such an important tool for self-care. Nurses do not provide nursing care in the absence of our own life experiences—understanding this and learning how to develop and enhance your own resilience are crucial.

In addition to an important focus on self-care, this new edition provides nurses with knowledge, skill, and strategies to help people move toward their own recovery. As we know, empowering people to be leaders in their own healthcare, regardless of the symptoms or challenges that they experience, can only have positive outcomes. This book provides the reader with strategies to enhance practice, and motivate, empower, and support a strength-focused approach with the people under their care as well as their families and communities. It provides clear and relevant chapters, discussing not only the theories that lay behind resilience but practical strategies to consider and use in the workplace and personally.

Mathematician, meteorologist, and theorist Edward Lorenz (2000) identified the notion that small events can have large, widespread consequences. The "butterfly effect" he described has become a metaphor for the existence of seemingly insignificant moments that alter history and shape destinies. Typically unrecognized at the time they occur, these moments create threads of cause and effect that appear obvious in retrospect, changing the course of a human life or rippling through the global economy. In this context, nursing work can at times look simple, but nurses—myself included—know it is not. We know there are flow-on effects to the work that we do every day that impact the lives of the people we come in contact with, as well as the lives of their families and communities. This book takes you on a journey to look beneath some of those interrelationships and explores strategies for all people—identifying how nurses can be leading change agents in the world of healthcare, one small step at a time.

It is so pleasing that this book is being published at a time when healthcare can seem so complicated and difficult—whether for the consumer or healthcare professionals. I commend the editors and contributors for leading the way in such important work; small, meaningful changes and every act of kindness, care, and compassion can have effects that last a lifetime.

*Kim Ryan*, Credentialed Mental Health Nurse
Adjunct Associate Professor, University of Sydney, Australia
CEO, Australian College of Mental Health Nurses

## REFERENCE

Lorenz, E. (2000). The butterfly effect. In R. Abraham & Y. Ueda (Eds.), *The chaos avant-garde: Memories of the early days of chaos theory* (pp. 91–94). Singapore: World Scientific Publishing Company.

# Preface

Welcome to the second edition of the volume that began life as *The Resilient Nurse: Empowering Your Practice*, which was published in 2011. This new edition differs in many ways from the first and includes a majority of newly commissioned chapters and new authors. This was important, as the field of resilience has changed significantly since this book was first compiled. Furthermore, the first edition focused on the resilience strategies that nurses can implement to strengthen themselves. In this second edition, we extend this insight, adding information on what nurses can also do to strengthen and motivate patients with whom they work, and who may be susceptible to feeling helpless in the face of overwhelming stressors. We explain that resilience, therefore, has a double purpose for nurses—it is a tool for self-care as well as for supporting and building strengths within patients, families, and communities. In this last category, we include the community of nursing and the healthcare community more generally.

To Mahatma Gandhi, the Indian philosopher and leader, is attributed a famous quote charging his followers to, "Be the change you wish to see in this world," although this—much misquoted—phrase was only actually used by a teacher, Arleen Lorrance, in the 1970s (see Lorrance, 1974, p. 85). Although not exactly Gandhi's words, this simple, yet profound message reflects his ethos and drives the rationale for this book. That rationale is for nurses to clarify their purpose as change agents and implement strategies that promote health and well-being in patients, individual nurses, nursing as a profession, the healthcare system, and society. That sounds ambitious, but that is how Gandhi lived his life. He chose to object to injustice, but he did this thoughtfully and carefully. Like many great leaders, he used both words and actions to great effect. He was not only a great orator, but also an aspirational role model for many others. Although he experienced personal conflicts and pain, he believed in active peacemaking and that this could be used for the benefit of the world and all its peoples. For these reasons, one of Gandhi's enduring messages, and one which can be directly applied to nursing, is that the actions of each individual *can* make a difference, not only to the individual, but to all those with whom that individual comes in contact. For nurses, this means not only the patients (and family and friends) whose lives they touch, but also the other nurses he or she works with, the healthcare setting in which they work, and the entire healthcare service. Each nurse will also affect and influence others indirectly. People watch and learn from the nurses around them, and their lives may be transformed by a single encounter with a nurse.

Nursing involves complex work in global health systems that are themselves becoming increasingly multifaceted. While nurses can flourish in such systems, they can also suffer. If a nurse is not prepared for the emotional and cognitive labor involved with caring, then the work of nursing can become a burden, leading to stress, burnout, and neglectful care. If a nurse is not, moreover, prepared to call out poor practice and step up into a leadership role when necessary, the problems in healthcare systems will never be resolved and are likely to increase in severity and negative impact.

Wherever nurses go, they encounter loss and suffering. It is impossible not to be touched and sometimes hurt by this, but through understanding suffering and compassion; practicing self-awareness, self-care, mindfulness, and other reflective practices; and working to gain a sense of meaning and connectedness, nurses may be better able to care both for patients and for themselves. This is what we see as developing resilience practices.

Within this book, several workplace challenges are discussed, and a range of strategies are presented to assist in avoiding or resolving such challenges. This will allow readers to be more prepared for new, difficult, and challenging encounters. Rather than feeling powerless, readers can arm themselves with awareness and problem-solving strategies that will assist them in feeling more confident about being a positive influence in their workplaces and their chosen profession. As a result, readers will feel less self-doubt and less tentativeness and suffer less emotional distress.

The aim of this book is to assist nurses to cultivate qualities and use proven strategies to retain personal professional strength. For, in the scheme of things, nurses have shown time and again that they are a precious and vital resource for society. Nurses are the hand that reaches out to offer comfort and connection. Nurses are the voice that translates jargon into understanding. Nurses are the actors that transform crisis into coping. Nurses are, and ought to be, the leaders in humanizing healthcare. Moreover, nurses are not alone in this endeavor. Every other clinician is charged with the same responsibility to move beyond the technique, the clipboard, and the technology to be a better human being.

Despite other clinicians' skills and foci, nurses are the linchpins of health services. Nurses are the human face of health services, for when people think of hospitals, they think of nurses. When people think of care, they think of nurses. Therefore, when things go wrong in healthcare, when people are dehumanized or experience undue suffering, people look to nurses, their surrogate mothers or fathers, to look out for them, to take charge, and to bring back order and control. Thus, the nurse's place in the healthcare environment, individually and collectively, is not only important, it is therefore formative in shaping the healthcare landscape.

Nursing is not an easy career, and no one will be a leader at the very beginning of that journey, or all the time even in a leadership position, but with determination and some words of inspiration, found, we hope, within the pages of this book, the personal qualities that lead individuals to nursing will be developed into mature leadership skills.

This book is structured into two parts that will help the reader to develop resilience and to be empowered to make changes based on thought rather than on reaction.

**Chapter 1** introduces the concept of resilience—a response to adversity that requires psychological as well as social adaptive responses in order to release emotional tension and bounce back to a productive way of living and working.

**Chapter 2** considers the qualities of nurses in history who made an enduring difference to the world and, of course, to nursing.

**Chapter 3** explores the contemporary problems that exist globally and that challenge the resilience of patients and healthcare providers. That solutions have not yet been found means they have become wicked problems and it is these that nurses, as change agents, need to be prepared for and become armed with effective and creative solutions.

**Chapter 4** elaborates on the concept of a resilience standpoint that assists in working out how nurses can relate to and communicate with patients in more facilitative and empowering ways than would a traditionally focused illness care practitioner and to relate to self and other nurses in ways that are supporting and motivating. The chapter also explores communication theories that explain some of the sources of misunderstandings in the workplace and provides strategies that can be used to interact assertively and effectively.

**Chapter 5** looks at ethical thinking as an organizing framework to help nurses appraise situations with logic and reason and then to think through dilemmas that could otherwise cause distress.

**Chapter 6** focuses on psychological thought processes, particularly our tendency to appraise people and situations automatically, which can result in hasty judgments that are colored by prejudice, past experiences, or faulty logic. In order to think more positively about challenges that may present, we must be aware of such tendencies.

**Chapter 7** explores complex health needs of patients and the realization that, if nurses are to work collaboratively with patients, they need to articulate what a holistic or ecological view of health and well-being means. Patients are social beings, not just bodies with organs and systems that succumb to disease. Their health and well-being are impacted by, and promoted by, what is going on psychologically, socially, environmentally, spiritually, and politically.

**Chapter 8** explores the reality that challenges the resilience of patients and clinicians—that people are no longer patients of just one healthcare system and that, because people do have complex needs and medicine and healthcare have diversified into specialties, patients and nurses cross many borders.

**Chapter 9** examines the impact of severe stress and adversity on people and the novel strategies that can be put into place to restore resilience, health, and well-being.

**Chapter 10** reminds nurses that one of the basic systems in which they work, nursing and multidisciplinary teams, is often an unappreciated asset. Working in teams is a nursing reality and yet understanding how to make them work effectively is often taken for granted. By focusing on the dynamics of teams, this chapter reclaims team work, team leaders, and followers as a vital resilience strategy.

**Chapter 11** considers what happens after the working day is over, so that meaning is made of any adversity encountered. In this way, stress is processed and let go. The chapter explores different kinds of coping strategies, encouraging the discerning use of practices that will assist in living a healthy life where work and personal lives are in harmony.

**Chapter 12** provides examples of nurses who embody another potential source of resilience—leadership skills—so that qualities can be revealed and elaborated upon, internalized by readers, and shared widely with nursing colleagues.

**Chapter 13** brings the book to a close by discussing one further resilience strategy that promises to strengthen an individual nurse's commitment and purpose—the power of professional unity. United groups know that there is strength in numbers.

Each chapter includes a series of activities that are designed to encourage readers to contemplate key concepts raised about resilience and how they can be adapted and implemented to support patients' well-being as well as their own. We have also produced a companion to the book as a resource for nursing instructors. The companion, which draws upon the expertise of experienced educators from across the world, provides teacher-oriented activities, multiple-choice questions, and trigger questions that can be used in class or online to promote student reflection, stimulate discussion, and inspire learners to take effective action in their professional lives.

*Qualified instructors may obtain access to supplementary material (Instructor's Manual and PowerPoints) by emailing textbook@springerpub.com.*

Nursing is exciting, rewarding, and responsible work. Nurses bear witness to other people's pain and may even experience vicarious trauma. To emerge positively and grow from all of the challenges they face, all nurses need to draw on the special quality of resilience and assist in developing resilient workplaces and more resilient and sustainable health systems that can better deliver the highest standards of person-centered care.

*Margaret McAllister*
*Donna Lee Brien*

## REFERENCE

Lorrance, A. (1974). The love project. In R. D. Kellough (Ed.), *Developing priorities and a style: Selected readings in education for teachers and parents* (pp. 85–97). Sacramento: California State University.

## ACKNOWLEDGMENTS

We wish to acknowledge and thank the contributors to this volume whose hard work and commitment to the project made this book possible. This new edition involved much more than updating of existing chapters, and we offer a sincere and warm thank you to those contributors for the good-spirited way in which they embraced the collaborative nature of this project. A warm thank you too to Joseph Morita, commissioning editor at Springer Publishing Company, who supported this project from its inception.

We would like to also gratefully acknowledge our university— Central Queensland University in Australia—for supporting the research that has resulted in this volume and for believing in our collaboration. Special recognition goes to the School of Nursing, Midwifery and Social Sciences, the School of Education and the Arts, and the Centre for Regional Advancement in Learning, Equity, Access and Participation at Central Queensland University for their ongoing support of our joint research.

Thank you to our two editorial interns Jo French and Jacqueline Green, who joined this project at a late stage, but offered some useful editorial assistance on the final draft of the manuscript.

A heartfelt thank you is also due to the many colleagues, friends, and family members who have offered their encouragement while we have worked on this project and devoted our energies to it.

Finally, as editors we would each like to thank each other. We have collaborated on many projects and brought to this volume our dissimilar scholarly and creative backgrounds, diverse approaches and networks, and different skill sets. We continue to learn with, and from, each other; perhaps because of this, working together has been one of the enriching pleasures of this project and, we both believe, at the heart of its realization.

# 1

# Resilience in Nursing

## Margaret McAllister and Donna Lee Brien

### INTRODUCTION

Nursing involves complex caring work—nurses support patients physically as well as mentally. During critical times of illness, patients may be vulnerable to stress buildup and breakdown, unless they are able to access and use effective strategies to avoid, reframe, or relieve negative stressors. At these times, nurses themselves may be vulnerable to the negative stressors by association. Witnessing other peoples' adversity can be traumatizing. Thus, the issues to be discussed in this chapter, the concept of resilience and how it can be developed, are relevant for nurses in two ways. Nurses can draw on knowledge about resilience to assist and encourage patients to withstand the pressures of ill health and to maximize their own strengths and supports to stay strong. Nurses can also apply what they know to their own health and well-being so that the physical, emotional, and cognitive labor involved with caring does not become a burden and deplete caring reserves.

The skill with which resilience strategies can be applied by nurses in their interactions with patients can be subtle and effective, yet when missing from care can leave patients feeling helpless and exposed.

## Donna's Story

Donna is in her late 50s and, after decades of good health, recently found herself in hospital having a major surgery. At the time of her operation, Donna was working as a senior academic in an Australian university in creative writing. Over the past 2 or 3 years, she had felt increasing pain in her groin, developed a pronounced limp when she walked, and had a decreasing scope of movement in her right hip. Neither over-the-counter nor prescription analgesics offered much relief. After numerous x-rays and scans, she was diagnosed as requiring a total hip replacement. This was very new for Donna. It was the first surgery she had needed since having her tonsils removed as a little girl. Her doctor recommended two local specialist surgeons and, after meeting them both, she was happy with her choice. The private hospital was conveniently nearby and had an excellent reputation. Donna had checked online for any issues with care and mishaps during surgery and was pleased to find news articles lauding her surgeon's ability. She also spoke with a number of friends and colleagues who all spoke highly of both the hospital and these doctors. She followed all the preoperative directions carefully and felt she had prepared as well as she could for the surgery, although she was, she admitted to her closest friends, quite fearful of the procedure and, especially, the anesthetic.

The joint replacement surgery went well, and after the surgery Donna received excellent care from many nurses, but one particular encounter was distressing. Although she was soon up and walking, Donna felt very nauseous, so much so that she was diagnosed as at least very sensitive to (if not allergic to) opiate-based pain killers. As a result, she was provided with an electric version of an ice pack that circulated cold water through a pad that, when left pressed against the area of the wound, significantly reduced her pain. This allowed Donna to reduce her analgesic intake and was very effective as long as the tub of ice water was replaced whenever it warmed up. Most nurses checked its function and quickly replaced it if Donna mentioned it needed to be, but there was one nurse who rolled her eyes and said, "You don't really need that anymore do you?" and removed the pad from Donna's hip. While she was doing so, she looked at the cover of the popular crime novel Donna was reading and sniffed, "I wouldn't have thought *you* would be reading *that* kind of book."

The nurse then swept out of the room with the apparatus, making sure Donna also knew how busy and short staffed the ward was that day. Donna felt the pain returning to the wound and endured it for an hour or so. When the operated-on area felt very hot and sore, she rang her buzzer, but the same nurse came into the room and asked, quite cuttingly, "And what do you think you need now, Professor?" Donna felt completely crushed and asked for some water. When the nurse had left, she tried to rest the cool glass against her hip, but it could not provide anything like the relief the ice pack had given her. She began to cry, and when a student nurse came in to check her blood pressure, she asked Donna what was wrong. When Donna mentioned her pain and continued nausea, the student retrieved the ice pack and asked another nurse to come and see Donna; this nurse dispensed some medication to help relieve the nausea. When Donna later thanked the student nurse and explained that one of the other nurses had taken the ice pack away, the student admitted that not all of the nursing team were on board with the new treatment.

Later that evening, Donna was confiding with her friend, a nursing professional, about her ordeal—her pain, the tension that arose because of the inconsistent care, and the mean-spiritedness of one of the most senior nurses. Her friend admitted that some older staff, although more experienced, were dismissive of complementary approaches to pain relief, thinking them inferior to analgesics, much more time-consuming to apply, and nothing more than new-age nonsense. They both noted the student nurse's attention and how much she had helped her patient.

## Learning From Donna's Story

This is our own story of a recent healthcare experience. Elements within the story reflect empowered actions on the part of the patient—she took charge, for example, of finding out about her surgical staff and the hospital. It is also a powerful example of the foreseen and unforeseen stressors that added to the illness experience culminating in a tipping point where Donna's self-caring resources were exhausted, and she was vulnerable to trauma. One nurse's demeanor and behavior eroded the patient's confidence to the point where she could not even ask for the care she knew she needed, and another's built it back up again in two actions that took, at maximum, 10 minutes. It is not clear how, or if, the nurses in the story consciously used resilience strategies in their interaction with the patient. It is also unclear whether they thought to apply resilience to their own work role. That there was tension between nurses, however slight, was evident, and if unaddressed, this could become draining and unproductive—and could even escalate. As a source of negative stress, peer tension can accumulate and one day it too could culminate in a tipping point for the student, who may decide that her ideals for practice are not shared by others and her commitment to nursing will fade. But what if that student were to develop positive communication strategies to reduce the tension, to clarify purpose, and to create a healthy workplace where patient comfort, well-being, and confidence remain a topmost priority?

The story reveals the simple things that patients and nurses can each do to foster their resilience. But it also reveals how nursing, like all other human service work, can be both taxing and rewarding. The purpose of this book is to maximize the strategies to make nursing work satisfying, effective, and empowering.

*The story reveals the simple things patients and nurses can each do to foster their resilience.*

## STRESS AND THE IMPORTANCE OF RESILIENCE

### Expectations of Today's Nurses

Being prepared for the challenges ahead may make all the difference in being able to persevere in your career and make a success of it. An important element to consider is what employers may expect from you. As a nurse in the 21st century, it is likely that your expectations and needs as a worker differ from those of previous generations. Unfortunately, the large bureaucracies, characteristic of many health services, can be slow to respond to changing needs (Hodges, Keeley, & Grier, 2005)—whether needs of patients, or the workforce. Holmes (2006) has described several characteristics typical of today's millennial workers and Glass (2007) adds some additional characteristics (Box 1.1).

**BOX 1.1  Characteristics of the Y Generation (Also Known as the Millennials)**

- Likely to have received a full high school education
- Envision many careers during their lifetime
- Technology-rich and multimedia literate
- Time-poor
- Impatient
- High expectations of employers:
  - Expect autonomy in the job
  - Less acceptance of seniority
  - Expect performance-based remuneration
  - Oriented toward results
- Need to see meaning and value in their workplace contributions
- Value work–life balance
- Unlikely to have loyalty to one employer

*Source:* Adapted from Glass, A. (2007). Understanding generational differences for competitive success. *Industrial and Commercial Training, 39*(2), 98–103. doi:10.1108/00197850710732424; Holmes, C. (2006). The slow death of psychiatric nursing: What next? *Journal of Psychiatric and Mental Health Nursing, 13*(4), 401–415. doi:10.1111/j.1365-2850.2006.00998.x.

If we add some of the negative characteristics of the typical health bureaucracy (Box 1.2), then we have the perfect recipe for conflict, stress, burnout, and neglectful care (Holmes, 2006).

*Being prepared for the challenges ahead may make all the difference in preventing undue stress, enjoying your work, and increasing success.*

Perhaps this is why some progressive health services are now instituting employee-friendly policies and practices and marketing themselves as great places to work (Figure 1.1).

## BOX 1.2  Negative Features of Large Bureaucracies

- Uneven staff skill mix
- Rapid staff turnover and instability
- Work conditions are employer focused
- Economics is the bottom line (consequences include widespread unpaid overtime)
- Rigid and disparaging management
- Controlling (leading to limited worker autonomy)

*Source:* Adapted from Holmes, C. (2006). The slow death of psychiatric nursing: What next? *Journal of Psychiatric and Mental Health Nursing, 13*(4), 401–415. doi:10.1111/j.1365-2850.2006.00998.x.

### Sources of Stress

Aside from having to work in a bureaucracy, sources of stress in nursing work are numerous. Rising patient acuity, rapid assessments and discharges, and increased service use by clients mean that nurses are dealing with sicker people who are likely to have multiple conditions that may complicate both the treatment and the recovery (Gaynor, Gattasch, Yorkston, Stewart, & Turner, 2006). These pressures can lead to work-role overload and burnout.

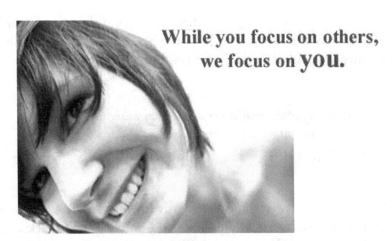

**Figure 1.1** Advertisement for recruiting nurses.

Therefore, the health service that you join is unlikely to be the comfortable, predictable, friendly place that is depicted in some television shows and prevalent in the public imagination. For a start, the people in teams will probably change quite rapidly. Certainly, the client turnaround will be fast. You may be quite regularly rostered to new areas to fill workforce gaps. Hence, understanding more about stress, and ways to reduce, manage, or overcome it, will be an important asset.

*Understanding more about stress will be an important asset to your career.*

In the mid-20th century, psychology involved the study of the individual human brain, particularly the abnormal brain. It was concerned about causes and treatments of disorders and tended to be preoccupied with a deficit approach. In practical terms, what this meant was that abnormal psychology was given far more emphasis than normal psychology. Stress became synonymous with distress and trauma. It was thought that stress was something that was always to be avoided. Occasionally, there might occur some individuals who appeared to be invulnerable to stress and they became an object of curiosity and hypothesizing. These resilient individuals were thought to be the bearers of a number of enviable traits, such as being naturally "stress-hardy" (Kobasa, 1982). Research in this era concentrated on identifying these traits so that they could be enhanced, and psychologists encouraged people to avoid the noxious effects of stress.

As time has gone on, psychology has undergone somewhat of a paradigm shift. The positive psychology movement (Seligman, 1998), with its interest in strengths and well-being, has broadened the examination of stress and its harmful effects to also include an appreciation for the useful effects of stress. Now we know that not all stress is bad. Some stress can be motivating and indeed enhance performance (Howells & Fletcher, 2015). This kind of stress is called *eustress* and could include things like going on a holiday, starting a new job, having a child, or retiring (Selye, 1976). Stressors like these are likely to be positively valued, may cause temporary anxiety but will also result in a sense of accomplishment and are positively reinforcing. The more we face them, the more we like them.

Also, we now know that stress buildup and breakdown does not just occur for vulnerable people like patients or at-risk communities. It also occurs in occupations that are dynamic, fast-paced, and involve being a witness to tragedy, trauma, or moral dilemmas, such as the military, doctors, nurses, paramedics, and police officers (Howe, Smajdor, & Stockl, 2012).

Another important development in thinking that has come from psychology is that people are capable of psychological growth and making positive change even *after* they have been hurt by trauma. This is called *posttraumatic growth* (Calhoun & Tedeschi, 2014). In addition, neurobiological research into the human brain has revealed that neural circuits can be shaped by adversity, and because these brain cells demonstrate *neuroplasticity* and can regenerate, strategies such as cognitive therapy, mindfulness, and meditation may be helpful in retraining the brain to rebound, recover, and change (Davidson & McEwen, 2012).

## The Stress Diathesis Model

The stress diathesis model suggests that accumulation of stress can lead to health breakdown (Figure 1.2). The model also proposes that people must first have a biological, psychological, or sociocultural predisposition to such disorders and must then be subjected to an immediate stressor to develop disease or other abnormality (Fontaine & Fletcher, 2003).

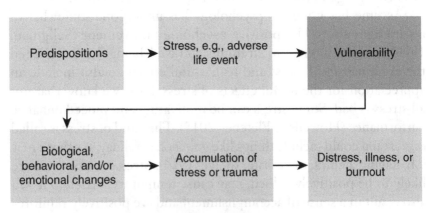

**Figure 1.2** The stress diathesis model.

Most people go through life with predispositions to various disorders that are never expressed. What protects them from succumbing to the stressor, or what methods they use to moderate that stressor, are important to understand and underscore the significance of another important and now quite widely discussed concept—*resilience*.

Put simply, resilience is a phenomenon of positive adjustment in the face of adversity (Masten & Powell, 2003). Research into resilience has been going on for over 50 years and has now achieved greater clarity in differentiating resilience from other human phenomena, such as stress-hardiness and strength of character or actions such as coping and surviving. Being precise about the definition of resilience is important, particularly for researchers and educators, because having a clear meaning about the term influences what resilience interventions should comprise and what scales to measure resilience should contain. When researchers are all using the same definition and measuring the same phenomenon, systematic improvements in the resilience of clients and nurses can occur. A common language about resilience is important to achieve.

## Evolution of the Concept of Resilience

Although the concept of resilience dates back to the 1800s, it was not until the 1970s that work on resilience expanded (Luthar, Cicchetti, & Becker, 2000). This was essentially due to the rise of psychology as a discipline. Initially, research was undertaken to explore a phenomenon seen in some children of parents diagnosed with schizophrenia who seemed to be thriving despite the adverse environment (Billings & Moos, 1983). The hypothesis emerged about there being a group of people who were *invincible* despite being *vulnerable* (Werner & Smith, 1982). Interest focused on the kinds of internal, psychological attributes that helped them survive ordeals. The work of Friborg, Barlaug, Martinussen, Rosenvinge, and Hjemdal (2005) identified four main psychological factors in such children: internal locus of control, optimism, bounce back, and stress-hardiness. An internal locus of control involves acknowledging one's own part in resolving challenges. In stressful periods, resilient individuals can use these attributes to bounce back and look forward.

Further studies have looked at marginalized children and adolescents who had experienced low socioeconomic circumstances, abuse, parental mental and chronic illness, violent communities, or tragic life incidents to find out what helped the survivors do well (Garmezy, Masten, & Tellegen, 1984; Jacelon, 1997). These and other studies showed that there are events outside the individual that seem to protect individuals from being overwhelmed by stress and became known as *protective factors*. Young people are likely to be able to deal with and overcome adversity better and are able to envision a future for themselves when there is *social connection* with family, peers, and other adults; when there is positive *role modeling* of winners or achievers; when there is unobtrusive *monitoring* of their well-being; and when there is *coaching* to help set goals and elevate expectations (Sroufe, Egeland, Carlson, & Collins, 2005).

Meanwhile, ecology researchers developed an interest in resilience by exploring an eco-system's capacity to absorb shocks and still maintain function (Folke, 2006). As concerns for sustainable environments increased, researchers began to identify and explore factors within a system that gave it capacity for renewal, reorganization, and development.

Research into resilience has since extended to adults. For example, research on people with schizophrenia ascertained that those with less severe symptoms were more likely to have positive outcomes in the areas of employment, responsibilities, and social relations, including marriage (Luthar et al., 2000). There have been studies on adults who survived childhood experiences of abuse and neglect but still managed to thrive in later life (Ben-David & Jonson-Reid, 2017). Similarly, survivors of domestic and family violence who turned their lives around (Dube & Rishi, 2017), people who live well despite AIDS (Fang et al., 2015) or cancer (Rowland & Baker, 2005), and people who endured terrorist attacks and natural disasters (Butler et al., 2005; Chang & Shinozuka, 2004) have demonstrated that succumbing to adversity is not inevitable. Insights from this work supported the justification of mental health interventions that targeted social and occupational factors *in addition to* symptom management.

The research also prompted thinking on factors to support well-being and productivity in other groups. A paradigm shift for health practitioners had begun. Antonovsky's (1987) concept of Sense of Coherence, which is influential in the public health discipline, is an example. In terms of this concept, a person's ability to cope in times of stress depends on three factors: meaningfulness, manageability, and comprehensibility. Meaningfulness is the profound experience that this stressor makes sense in one's life and thus coping is desirable; manageability is the recognition of the resources required to meet the demands of the situation and a willingness to search them out; and comprehensibility is the perception of the world as being understandable, meaningful, orderly, and consistent, rather than chaotic, random, and unpredictable.

Thus, continued research investigations in psychology, psychiatry, nursing, occupational therapy, health promotion, and sports science have shown the limitations of a deficit model that only examines problems as a result of stress and have deepened appreciation for the role that health and well-being have for individuals and societies. Thanks to this multidisciplinary lens now being trained on resilience, resilience-building has shifted from a narrow focus as a remedial measure to reduce stress and anxiety, to a broader focus on capacity building to enable people, teams, and organizations to sustain high levels of performance in challenging circumstances.

Currently, there is widespread agreement that human resilience involves being able to access psychological as well as social resources, and three levels of protective factors: individual, family, and community (see Table 1.1).

Table 1.1 Resilience Resources at Individual, Family, and Social/ Environment Levels

| Resources | Protective Strategy |
| --- | --- |
| **Individual** | |
| *Psychological* | Positive temperament |
| | Robust neurobiology |
| *Social* | Responsiveness to others |
| | Prosocial attitudes |
| | Attachment to others |
| *Intelligence* | Academic achievement |
| | Planning and decision-making |

(continued)

**Table 1.1** Resilience Resources at Individual, Family, and Social/Environment Levels (*continued*)

| Resources | Protective Strategy |
| --- | --- |
| *Communication skills* | Developed language |
| | Advanced reading |
| *Personal attributes* | Tolerance for negative affect |
| | Self-efficacy and esteem |
| | Internal locus of control |
| | Sense of humor |
| | Hopefulness |
| | Strategies to deal with stress |
| | Enduring set of values |
| | Balanced perspective on experience |
| | Malleability and flexibility |
| | Fortitude, conviction, tenacity, and resolve |
| **Family level** | |
| *Supportive families* | Parental warmth, encouragement, and assistance |
| | Cohesion and care within the family |
| | Close relationship with a caring adult |
| | Belief in the child |
| | Nonblaming |
| | Marital support |
| | Talent or hobby valued by others |
| *Socioeconomic status* | Material resources |
| **Community level** | |
| *School experiences* | Supportive peers |
| | Positive teacher influences |
| | Success (academic or other) |
| *Supportive communities* | Belief in the individual |
| | Nonpunitive |

(*continued*)

Table 1.1 Resilience Resources at Individual, Family, and Social/
Environment Levels (continued)

| Resources | Protective Strategy |
| --- | --- |
| | Provisions and resources to assist belief in the values of society |
| Cultural resources | Traditional activities |
| | Traditional spirituality |
| | Traditional languages |
| | Traditional healing |

Source: Adapted from Olsson, C., Bond, L., Burns, J. M., Vella-Broderick, D. A., & Sawyer, S. M. (2003). Adolescent resilience: A concept analysis. Journal of Adolescence, 26, 1–11. doi:10.1016/s0140-1971(02)00118-5.

Based on all of this research, we now know that resilience does not only concern a person's psychological or internal makeup. Resilience is not only about the way one appraises a situation (whether it is perceived as "a horrendous ordeal" or "a challenge to be surmounted"). It is also not about what the individual can personally do to change, but a shared social responsibility. Social actions, such as lending support, being a sounding board, and offering role models to inspire perseverance and a positive attitude can be effective in supporting resilience. In short, resilience is a combination of these elements. Two definitions are illuminating for nurses because one focuses on patient care and the other takes a more structural approach. They are:

1. Resilience is a constellation of characteristics that protect individuals from the potential negative effect of stressors. (Fletcher & Sarkar, 2012)
2. Resilience is the capacity of a system to use shocks and disturbances—to spur renewal and innovative thinking. (Stockholm Resilience Centre, 2016, p. 3)

These insights have supported mental health interventions that targeted social and occupational factors, in addition to symptom management. They also prompted thinking on what factors could support well-being and productivity in other groups. As a result, a paradigm shift began for health practitioners. For many, this has meant a reorientation from a concern focused on illness to also considering well-being and how to foster it.

## Looking at Survivors to Develop a Science of Well-Being

Aaron Antonovsky (1987) introduced the term *salutogenesis* to describe the support of health and well-being rather than a focus on the factors that cause disease. The concept has influenced public health (Gregg & O'Hara, 2007), psychology (Suedfeld, 2005), healthy aging (Wiesmann & Hannich, 2010), and nursing and midwifery (Cuellar & Zaiontz, 2012; Perez-Botella, Downe, Magistretti, Lindstrom, & Berg, 2015; Stock, 2017). It has also been applied to the workplace and organizations, and their design and management (Bauer & Jenny, 2013; Nilsson, Andersson, Ejlertsson, & Troein, 2012).

The term *salutogenesis* comes from the Latin, *salus* meaning health and the Greek, *genesis* meaning origin. Antonovsky studied the influence of various stressors on health and was able to show that relatively unstressed people had much more resistance to illness than those who were more stressed. In his analysis, Antonovsky argued that the experience of well-being constitutes a *sense of coherence*. He defined this as, "a pervasive, enduring though dynamic feeling of confidence that one's internal and external environments are predictable and that there is a high probability that things will work out as well as can reasonably be expected" (Antonovsky, 1979, p. 123). We might understand this as believing the world is a rational place and approaching this with an optimistic and positive outlook.

Smith (2002) suggested that a strong sense of coherence assists a person's ability to cope and consists of three factors: meaningfulness—understanding that this stressor makes sense in one's life and, thus, coping is desirable; manageability—the recognition that there are resources required to meet the demands of the situation and a willingness to search out those resources; and comprehensibility—the perception of the world as understandable, meaningful, and orderly and consistent rather than chaotic, random, and unpredictable.

Survivor stories, mostly told in the form of personal memoirs, are today a recognized genre of literature and read by many. Narratives by those who survived the Holocaust such as Elie Wiesel (1958),

Viktor Frankl (1963), and Primo Levi (1979) have inspired work in psychotherapy, philosophy, peace studies, and literature. Frankl, for example, emerged from the Holocaust without the deep emotional injuries found in many survivors of the Nazi death camps. His compassion for his fellow prisoners led him to want to develop ways to help them maintain their will to live. In fact, this terrible experience ultimately enriched Frankl's life and that of many others. Thus, the long-term consequences of even such unimaginable extreme trauma may include increased personal strength and growth. This phenomenon, now known as *posttraumatic growth*, is a growing area of research within psychology and psychiatry (Calhoun & Tedeschi, 2014; Linley & Joseph, 2004; Tedeschi & Calhoun, 2004).

Primo Levi wrote an influential book on the ability of the human spirit to rise above suffering. This volume has been motivating and inspirational to many who have needed courage to endure. Similarly, Elie Wiesel's famous statement "to remain silent and indifferent is the greatest sin of all" was his life motto as he pursued a lifelong commitment to world peace. In 1986, this was recognized when he was awarded the Nobel Peace Prize. Another example of thriving through adversity is the story of Lt. Commander Charlie Plumb (1995). Plumb was a navy pilot shot down early in the Vietnam War. He was taken to a prison in Hanoi and kept in a stone cell for 6 years, where he was tortured and deprived. He said of that experience, "It's probably the most valuable 6 years of my life. Amazing what a little adversity can teach a person. I really felt there was some meaning to that, to my experience itself" (quoted in Siebert, 1996, p. 6). Many other examples can be found in the memoirs that people have written as survivors of various illnesses, abuses, bereavement, or other adverse situations. Segal (1986) summarizes the significance of this survivor research thus:

> Those who have suffered and prevail find that after their ordeal they begin to operate at a higher level than ever before. . . . The terrible experiences of our lives, despite the pain they bring, may become our redemption. (p. 130)

This survivor-focused research has relevance to the processes of building resilience in health professionals. Evocative, moving stories from survivors about their experiences can contribute to others' learning by enhancing awareness of the power of the human spirit to endure and overcome and by revealing the value of generative practices such as concern and altruism. Using storytelling may also be a powerful and effective way to "inoculate" students of the health profession against future stress and burnout by raising their awareness of resilience strategies and providing them with examples of how to transcend adversity (McAllister & McKinnon, 2009).

## Positive Appraisal of Stressors, Coping, and Transcendence

Although psychological assets are only part of the picture for resilience, it is important that individuals learn how to maximize their own capacity to moderate stress and cope with life's challenges. The internal or psychological traits of resilience are termed "resiliency." Whether we see a stressor as good or bad, leading to eustress or distress, depends on our cognitive appraisal of the situation. This concept is explored more fully in Chapter 6, Appraising and Moderating Stressful Situations.

Research has produced new thinking on how we can develop good, or adaptive, coping skills to manage stress (Holton, Barry, & Chaney, 2016). Essentially, there are three broad categories of coping strategies (Table 1.2).

As well as how we personally adapt to the situation, there are social strategies that may enhance or impede our resilience. How the family functions and supports each other, whether a person is active or passive in the ways they cope, are all strategies and predictors for

| Table 1.2 Three Types of Coping Strategies | |
| --- | --- |
| Problem focused | Approach strategies such as seeking support; situation control, such as limiting other stressors; make positive self-statements |
| Emotion focused | Minimization, short-term avoidance, cognitive restructuring—"it will teach me something," positive reframe |
| Maladaptive | Denial, numbing (substance use), avoidance, disengagement, rumination, resignation, venting/displacement, aggression (this can be inter-group; patient/nurse; and cyclical) |

how well we are likely to adapt to stress such as illness and adversity in our lives. Adaptive coping strategies can be applied across the life span and thus nurses need a good understanding for how they might facilitate coping in childhood through to old age. Mullins et al. (2015), for instance, found that an intervention that focused on decreasing parent distress associated with uncertainty over their child's illness and treatment improved the child's adaptation to cancer. In another study, McAllister, Knight, and Withyman (2017) found that engaging early high school students in imaginative discussion-based activities about the challenges of adolescence extended their coping repertoire. The intervention in this study focused on exposing participants to role models who were winners in challenging scenarios, able to transform conflict into turning points, and active peacemakers. In older adults, too, resilience work is flourishing. For example, interventions that encourage and develop "self-transcendence," which involves a sense of connectedness between a person and the wider world, and a reflection on the ways stress has been accepted or accommodated in his or her life, has shown positive impact on the resilience of older people (Haugan, 2014; Teixeira, 2008).

### Resilience May Involve Context-Specific Skills

Psychology no longer exclusively focuses on individuals and the inner workings of their brain. Now they acknowledge that individuals are social beings and their strengths and vulnerabilities can be shaped by their surroundings. Structural factors in society, such as entrenched poverty or advantage, can have an effect on whether a person will be resilient or break down (Metzl & Hansen, 2014). Similarly, problems in the social world may not be simply *a fact of life* that needs to be coped with, but perhaps seen as an issue that needs to be changed. No longer are clinicians preoccupied with deficit models of care (Windle, Bennett, & Noyes, 2011). Deficit models are those that focus on problems and deficiencies, and clinical interventions tend to focus on repairing the problem. But such an approach tends to be reactive and not proactive. It also does not involve the client in actively engaging in healthy living and maximizing their own strengths and potential.

Another view of resilience is the notion that resilience is contextual and dynamic (Gu & Day, 2007). That is, individuals may not display resilience in all aspects of their lives, and various life transitions may activate different genetically determined biological reactions that require different coping mechanisms, social supports, and spiritual

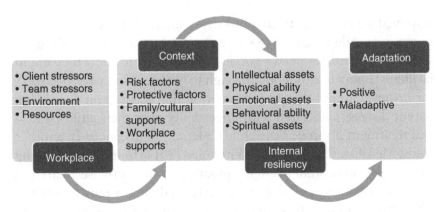

**Figure 1.3** A dynamic framework of resilience.

strength. In addition, some resilience resources that individuals possess may be readily available in some contexts but not in others. For example, social supports may be forthcoming in situations that involve publicly acknowledged crises. However, when a crisis is associated with a situation that brings stigma or shame to a person, then supports may not be accessible, and maintaining resilience may require coping of a different magnitude or quality (Deveson, 2003). Seen from this viewpoint, resilience has an added contextual dimension involving an interaction among the stressor, the context, and personal characteristics (Figure 1.3).

### Resilience Across Cultures and Communities

Resilience has also been viewed as a complex cultural construct that involves a dynamic interaction between an individual and the family, with the maintenance of positive adaptation occurring despite adverse experiences (Walsh, 2015). This viewpoint notably includes the concept of the family as an entity that can possess a group resilience, rather than only individuals demonstrating resilience.

Across cultures, similar factors have been found to contribute to resilience. Lothe and Heggen (2003), for instance, found resilience in survivors of the Ethiopian famine of 1984–1985. These survivors commonly demonstrated faith, hope, and valued memories of their homeland.

Through the study of vulnerable cultures and communities, there is now an increased knowledge about community resilience, that is, the ability of a community to deal with adversity and in so doing, reach a higher level of functioning. Hallett, Chandler, and Lalonde (2007), for example, found that North American aboriginal communities with the following features tended to be more resilient: self-government, land claims, education, health services, cultural facilities, police and fire, and use of own language. Numerous researchers have found that cultural identification or attachment and communities that build positive self-image improve these groups' resilience (Hegney, Eley, Plank, Buikstra, & Parker, 2006). If they work on reducing risk factors and breaking any negative cycles, resilience also grows. In indigenous communities, there are two main risk factors: discrimination and historical trauma that involves unresolved grief (Fleming & Ledogar, 2008). Specific risks that occur in a community, such as drug misuse may compound these primary risks.

This notion of attachment and positive identity is equally relevant to health practitioners who operate as a community, and within communities.

*Resilient communities transcend adversity because members feel bonded to each other and to the community.*

### Resilience at Work

The knowledge gained from research into resilient communities has also been applied to communities of workers, such as nurses, because it is not just vulnerable or ill individuals who experience adversity and need resilience—the well-being of workers is also important.

The resilience of workers, like the resilience of vulnerable communities, is currently under threat because of several issues, including the pressures of austerity policies. When the global financial crisis occurred in 2008, many nations' governments severely tightened their welfare spending and put a freeze on wage rises. Since this time workplace conditions have gradually deteriorated so that workers are expected to do more, with fewer rewards. In healthcare, austerity policies mean that problems such as short-staffing, uneven skill mixes, wage-freezing, casualization, violence, bullying, and burnout have festered and created a situation where workers feel distressed, angry, or unfulfilled and are not working to their fullest capacity (Schrecker, 2016).

Even without the pressure of tight policy constraints, the health environment is stressful, making it highly likely that clinicians will experience workplace adversity. Hunter and Warren (2014), for example, found that in the UK midwives are experiencing rising levels of adversity because of a constellation of factors: the unabating national shortage of midwives, rising birth rates, and increased numbers of women presenting with complex care needs. The impact of this adversity on individual midwives and the profession is significant—low morale, increased sickness, and high attrition rates feed into a cycle of dissatisfaction and workforce churn, itself putting more pressure on already overworked midwives. Studies have repeatedly found that nurses and other healthcare workers are vulnerable to stress breakdown, which seriously affects processes and outcomes in health systems (Aiken, Clarke, Sloane, Lake, & Cheney, 2008; Khamisa, Oldenburg, Peltzer, & Ilic, 2015; Schaufeli, Leiter, & Maslach, 2009).

Consequently, in the last decade, workplace resilience interventions have flourished (Foster et al., 2018; Mehta et al., 2016; Pipe et al., 2012; Sull, Harland, & Moore, 2015). In a systematic review of workplace resilience, Robertson, Cooper, Sarkar, and Curran (2015) found that successful programs were those that used a range of strategies. These include: (a) realistic simulations of adverse conditions so that participants could be exposed to relevant stressful incidents, (b) rehearsal of ways of confronting and moderating the associated emotional and physical pressures, and (c) transforming the way stress is perceived and managed.

Robertson et al. (2015) found that several cognitive rehearsal techniques were effective in promoting clarity of thought. These were mindfulness, meditation, and self-compassion to assist in calming anxiety, self-talk to allow self-regulation, and assist in problem-solving. Another useful inclusion in these interventions is to provide coaches who model coping and an optimistic outlook, reframe stressors, and support people to keep focused on goals, bounce back from any critical stressors, and attain success. It is also important to include opportunities for participants to reflect on practice so that actions taken can be reviewed and revised. Finally, workplace resilience requires a combination of interventions focused on the individual and the community. Thus, personal support strategies as well as strategies to foster a healthy workplace culture are vital (King, Newman, & Luthans, 2016).

Ongoing interest in resilience in the workplace has led to an agreement that resilience is a capacity that can develop over time in the context of person-environment interactions.

*Healthy work environments have the capacity to improve overall health and well-being of the workers.*

## Relevance of Resilience Research to Nursing

Resilience research presents some important concepts that are readily applicable to nurses. Most of the literature divides resilience into factors that either protect people or put them at risk. Protective factors such as positive coping mechanisms and the ability to harness and use social supports and personal spirituality, which are known to help children, youth, older people, and those surviving traumatic experiences, are readily applicable to nurses. Moreover, evidence suggests that these positive qualities may be developed through learning experiences. Some of the risk factors that have been identified in groups such as soldiers, prisoners of war, and displaced or traumatized people may also be directly applicable to nurses. However, exploratory and intervention-based research to examine resilience as a tool for dealing with stress in healthcare workplaces is only just beginning, and there is much more to discover (Gillespie, Chaboyer, & Wallis, 2009; Hegney, Rees, Eley, Osseiran-Moisson, & Francis, 2015; Slatyer et al., 2017).

An aspect of resilience often overlooked and certainly often ignored within the context of the health workplace is the action that can be taken and the changes implemented to moderate the impact of stress and adversity on workers' lives. This means that everyone should be proactive about resilience in the workplace. Healthcare work is always going to be busy, unpredictable, and emotionally demanding of clinicians, and so nurses need more than good defenses against stressful workplace cultures. They also need to receive support to develop positive strategies and outlooks, in such ways as via mentoring and education. Survivors of adversity show how this can be done. For people like Frankl, survival was not about being *helped* by others; it was about him searching for and locating something resourceful and sustaining deep within himself. Then, it was about him giving back to others in order to assist them through this process. This *generativity*, as demonstrated by Frankl's altruism, and his setting a good example, by mentoring, leading, coaching, and motivating others, is a practice that can be learned by, and strengthened in, those entering the health professions.

*Nurses need more than good coping mechanisms and should be proactive about resilience in the workplace.*

Furthermore, a *systems approach* to resilience may assist nurses to understand that change can be facilitated at many levels: with the client, the clinician, and the healthcare environment.

## CONCLUSION

Resilience is a complex combination of personal attributes, social actions, and learned strategies to protect a person or group from succumbing to the negative stress arising from adversity and trauma. Useful cognitive strategies that can be applied and learned include abilities to calm down and self-soothe, problem solve, transcend the difficulties, and replace judgment with compassion. Resilience does not involve simply accepting negative stress and minimizing it. Also, resilience in one aspect of our life may not necessarily mean that we will be resilient in other aspects. Resilience is contextual. Future-focused social strategies are also important in building resilience. These may include efforts to strengthen self and group identity, resolve any ongoing grief and loss issues, and adopt an outlook that crises can be viewed as a predictable disturbance in the system that to be rectified, requires confrontation, problem-solving, and an optimistic expectation. The system is unlikely to repair itself without creative solutions.

Understanding that the way individuals approach and view an event determines the outcome, rather than the event itself, is a powerful message to carry through one's career. Predictors of resilience such as cognitive ability, adaptability, positive self-identity, social support, coping skills, spiritual connection, the ability to find meaning in adversity, and generative skills are all qualities that can be learned or strengthened. Hence, *you* can do something about developing a patient's resilience as well as your own. As Donna's story suggests, the actions patients take to be active participants in their own healthcare are a vital yet sometimes hidden resilience resource. Nurses can search for and validate these with every person. Respect for a patient, attuned listening, validating self-care and coping strategies, and being responsive to a patient's needs are small acts that foster resilience. Ignoring stressors that occur for nurses may be one way to cope in a busy environment where values clash between peers, but it is not a long-term solution. Undercurrents of conflict that flow unabated can accumulate and culminate in trauma sometime in the future. This is why honest, respectful communication of values and ethics needs to be learned and enacted as an everyday resilience tactic. It can change the culture and put patients' needs first.

## TIPS

There are many healthy ways to manage and cope with stress.

You can either **change the situation** or **change your reaction**. As everyone has a unique response to stress, there is no "one-size-fits-all" solution to managing it. No single method works for everyone in every situation, so experiment with different techniques and strategies. Focus on what makes you feel calm and in control. This can be summarized as follows:

**Dealing With Stressful Situations: The Four As**

*Change the situation:*

- **Avoid** the stressor
- **Alter** the stressor

*Change your reaction:*

- **Adapt** to the stressor
- **Accept** the stressor

## LEARNING ACTIVITIES

1. Access the resilience inventory at http://www.resiliencescale .com/. Complete the test and then reflect on your strengths and your vulnerabilities. If you feel comfortable doing so, share these insights with your peers in a group discussion.

2. Make a table of Donna's strengths and vulnerabilities. In the left column, list the strengths she revealed that potentially supported her resilience. In the right column, list the things that occurred that eroded her resilience. Are there any nurse-initiated actions in either column?
3. What strategies could you suggest that the nurses engage in to reflect on how the care for patients such as Donna may be improved now that you have a fuller understanding of resilience and well-being?
4. How might these strategies be directed inwardly toward nurses and nursing?

## REFERENCES

Aiken, L. H., Clarke, S. P., Sloane, D. M., Lake, E. T., & Cheney, T. (2008). Effects of hospital care environment on patient mortality and nurse outcomes. *The Journal of Nursing Administration, 38*(5), 223. doi:10.1097/01.NNA.0000312773.42352.d7

Antonovsky, A. (1979). *Health, stress, and coping.* San Francisco, CA: Jossey-Bass.

Antonovsky, A. (1987). *Unraveling the mystery of health: How people manage stress and stay well.* San Francisco, CA: Jossey-Bass.

Bauer, G. F., & Jenny, G. J. (Eds.). (2013). *Salutogenic organizations and change: The concepts behind organizational health intervention research.* New York, NY: Springer.

Ben-David, V., & Jonson-Reid, M. (2017). Resilience among adult survivors of childhood neglect: A missing piece in the resilience literature. *Children and Youth Services Review, 78,* 93–103. doi:10.1016/j.childyouth.2017.05.014

Billings, A., & Moos, R. (1983). Comparisons of children of depressed and non-depressed parents: A social–environmental perspective. *Journal of Abnormal Child Psychology, 11*(4), 463–486. doi:10.1007/BF00917076

Butler, L., Blasey, C., Garlan, R., McCaslin, S., Azarow, J., Chen, X., . . . Spiegel, D. (2005). Posttraumatic growth following the terrorist attacks of September 11, 2001: Cognitive, coping, and trauma symptom predictors in an Internet convenience sample. *Traumatology, 11*(4), 247–267. doi:10.1177/153476560501100405

Calhoun, L. G., & Tedeschi, R. G. (Eds.). (2014). *Handbook of posttraumatic growth: Research and practice.* New York, NY: Psychology Press.

Chang, S. E., & Shinozuka, M. (2004). Measuring improvements in the disaster resilience of communities. *Earthquake Spectra, 20*(3), 739–755. doi:10.1193/1.1775796

Cuellar, E. H., & Zaiontz, R. G. (2012). Salutogenic nursing education: A summative review. *Journal of Nursing Education and Practice, 3*(5), 89. doi:10.5430/jnep.v3n5p89

Davidson, R. J., & McEwen, B. S. (2012). Social influences on neuroplasticity: Stress and interventions to promote well-being. *Nature Neuroscience, 15*(5), 689. doi:10.1038/nn.3093

Deveson, A. (2003). *Resilience.* Sydney, Australia: Penguin.

Dube, S. R., & Rishi, S. (2017). Utilizing the salutogenic paradigm to investigate well-being among adult survivors of childhood sexual abuse and other adversities. *Child Abuse & Neglect, 66,* 130–141. doi:10.1016/j.chiabu.2017.01.026

Fang, X., Vincent, W., Calabrese, S. K., Heckman, T. G., Sikkema, K. J., Humphries, D. L., & Hansen, N. B. (2015). Resilience, stress, and life quality in older adults living with HIV/AIDS. *Aging & Mental Health, 19*(11), 1015–1021. doi:10.10 80/13607863.2014.1003287

Fleming, J., & Ledogar, R. J. (2008). Resilience, an evolving concept: A review of literature relevant to Aboriginal research. *Pimatisiwin, 6*(2), 7.

Fletcher, D., & Sarkar, M. (2012). A grounded theory of psychological resilience in Olympic champions. *Psychology of Sport and Exercise, 13,* 669–678. doi:10.1016/j. psychsport.2012.04.007

Folke, C. (2006). Resilience: The emergence of a perspective for social–ecological systems analyses. *Global Environmental Change, 16*(3), 253–267. doi:10.1016/j. gloenvcha.2006.04.002

Fontaine, K., & Fletcher, S. (2003). *Mental health nursing* (5th ed.). Upper Saddle River, NJ: Pearson.

Foster, K., Schochet, I., Wurfl, A., Roche, M., Maybery, D., Shakespeare-Finch, J., & Furness, T. (2018). On PAR: A feasibility study of the Promoting Adult Resilience programme with mental health nurses. *International Journal of Mental Health Nursing, 27,* 1470–1480. doi:10.1111/inm.12447

Frankl, V. (1963). *Man's search for meaning.* New York, NY: Washington Square Press.

Friborg, O., Barlaug, D., Martinussen, M., Rosenvinge, J. H., & Hjemdal, O. (2005). Resilience in relation to personality and intelligence. *International Journal of Methods in Psychiatric Research, 14*(1), 29–42. doi:10.1002/mpr.15

Garmezy, N., Masten, A. S., & Tellegen, A. (1984). The study of stress and competence in children: A building block for developmental psychopathology. *Child Development, 55,* 97–111. doi:10.2307/1129837

Gaynor, L., Gattasch, T., Yorkston, E., Stewart, S., & Turner, C. (2006). Where do all the undergraduate and new graduate nurses go and why? A search for empirical research evidence. *Australian Journal of Advanced Nursing, 24*(2), 26–32.

Gillespie, B. M., Chaboyer, W., & Wallis, M. (2009). The influence of personal characteristics on the resilience of operating room nurses: A predictor study. *International Journal of Nursing Studies, 46*(7), 968–976. doi:10.1016/j. ijnurstu.2007.08.006

Glass, A. (2007). Understanding generational differences for competitive success. *Industrial and Commercial Training, 3*(2), 98–103. doi:10.1108/00197850 710732424

Gregg, J., & O'Hara, L. (2007). Values and principles evident in current health promotion practice. *Health Promotion Journal of Australia, 18*(1), 7–11. doi:10.1071/ HE07007

Gu, Q., & Day, C. (2007). Teachers' resilience: A necessary condition for effectiveness. *Teaching and Teacher Education, 23*(8), 1302–1316. doi:10.1016/j.tate.2006.06.006

Hallett, D., Chandler, M., & Lalonde, C. (2007). Aboriginal language knowledge and youth suicide. *Cognitive Development, 22,* 392–399. doi:10.1016/j.cogdev.2007.02.001

Haugan, G. (2014). Nurse–patient interaction is a resource for hope, meaning in life and self-transcendence in nursing home patients. *Scandinavian Journal of Caring Sciences, 28*(1), 74–88. doi:10.1111/scs.12028

Hegney, D., Eley, R., Plank, A., Buikstra, E., & Parker, V. (2006). Workforce issues in nursing in Queensland: 2001 and 2004. *Journal of Clinical Nursing, 15*(12), 1521–1530. doi:10.1111/j.1365-2702.2006.01558.x

Hegney, D. G., Rees, C. S., Eley, R., Osseiran-Moisson, R., & Francis, K. (2015). The contribution of individual psychological resilience in determining the professional quality of life of Australian nurses. *Frontiers of Psychology, 6,* 1613. doi:10.3389/fpsyg.2015.01613

Hodges, H. F., Keeley, A. C., & Grier, E. C. (2005). Professional resilience, practice longevity, and Parse's theory for baccalaureate education. *Journal of Nursing Education, 44*(12), 548–554. doi:10.3928/00220124-20190115-01

Holmes, C. (2006). The slow death of psychiatric nursing: What next? *Journal of Psychiatric and Mental Health Nursing, 13*(4), 401–415. doi:10.1111/j.1365-2850.2006.00998.x

Holton, M. K., Barry, A. E., & Chaney, J. D. (2016). Employee stress management: An examination of adaptive and maladaptive coping strategies on employee health. *Work, 53*(2), 299–305. doi:10.3233/WOR-152145

Howe, A., Smajdor, A., & Stöckl, A. (2012). Towards an understanding of resilience and its relevance to medical training. *Medical Education, 46*(4), 349–356. doi:10.1111/j.1365-2923.2011.04188.x

Howells, K., & Fletcher, D. (2015). Sink or swim: Adversity- and growth-related experiences in Olympic swimming champions. *Psychology of Sport and Exercise, 16,* 37–48. doi:10.1016/j.psychsport.2014.08.004

Hunter, B., & Warren, L. (2014). Midwives' experiences of workplace resilience. *Midwifery, 30*(8), 926–934. doi:10.1016/j.midw.2014.03.010

Jacelon, C. (1997). The trait and process of resilience. *Journal of Advanced Nursing, 25*(1), 123–129. doi:10.1046/j.1365-2648.1997.1997025123.x

Khamisa, N., Oldenburg, B., Peltzer, K., & Ilic, D. (2015). Work related stress, burnout, job satisfaction and general health of nurses. *International Journal of Environmental Research and Public Health, 12*(1), 652–666. doi:10.3390/ijerph120100652

King, D. D., Newman, A., & Luthans, F. (2016). Not if, but when we need resilience in the workplace. *Journal of Organizational Behavior, 37*(5), 782–786. doi:10.1002/job.2063

Kobasa, S. (1982). The hardy personality: Toward a social psychology of stress and health. *Social Psychology of Health and Illness, 4,* 3–32.

Levi, P. (1979). *If this is a man.* London, England: Penguin.

Linley, P. A., & Joseph, S. (2004). Positive change following trauma and adversity: A review. *Journal of Traumatic Stress, 17*(1), 11–21. doi:10.1023/B:JOTS.0000014671.27856.7e

Lothe, E., & Heggen, K. (2003). A study of resilience in young Ethiopian famine survivors. *Journal of Transcultural Nursing, 14*(4), 313–320. doi:10.1177/1043659603257161

Luthar, S., Cicchetti, D., & Becker, B. (2000). The construct of resilience: A critical evaluation and guidelines for future work. *Child Development, 27*(3), 543–562. doi:10.1111/1467-8624.00164

Masten, A., & Powell, J. (2003). A resilience framework for research, policy, and practice. In S. Luthar (Ed.), *Resilience and vulnerability: Adaptation in the context of childhood adversities*. New York, NY: Columbia University Press.

McAllister, M., Knight, B. A., & Withyman, C. (2017). Building resilience in regional youth: Impacts of a universal mental health promotion program. *International Journal of Mental Health Nursing, 27*(3), 1044–1054. doi:10.1111/inm.12412

McAllister, M., & McKinnon, J. (2009). The importance of teaching and learning resilience in the health disciplines: A critical review of the literature. *Nurse Education Today, 29*, 371–379. doi:10.1016/j.nedt.2008.10.011

Mehta, D. H., Perez, G. K., Traeger, L., Park, E. R., Goldman, R. E., Haime, V., . . . Jackson, V. A. (2016). Building resiliency in a palliative care team: A pilot study. *Journal of Pain and Symptom Management, 51*(3), 604–608. doi:10.1016/j.jpainsymman.2015.10.013

Metzl, J., & Hansen, H. (2014). Structural competency: Theorizing a new medical engagement with stigma and inequality. *Social Science and Medicine, 103*, 126–133. doi:10.1016/j.socscimed.2013.06.032

Mullins, L. L., Molzon, E. S., Suorsa, K. I., Tackett, A. P., Pai, A. L., & Chaney, J. M. (2015). Models of resilience: Developing psychosocial interventions for parents of children with chronic health conditions. *Family Relations, 64*(1), 176–189. doi:10.1111/fare.12104

Nilsson, P., Andersson, I. H., Ejlertsson, G., & Troein, M. (2012). Workplace health resources based on sense of coherence theory. *International Journal of Workplace Health Management, 5*(3), 156–167. doi:10.1108/17538351211268809

Perez-Botella, M., Downe, S., Magistretti, C. M., Lindstrom, B., & Berg, M. (2015). The use of salutogenesis theory in empirical studies of maternity care for healthy mothers and babies. *Sexual & Reproductive Healthcare, 6*(1), 33–39. doi:10.1016/j.srhc.2014.09.001

Pipe, T. B., Buchda, V. L., Launder, S., Hudak, B., Hulvey, L., Karns, K. E., & Pendergast, D. (2012). Building personal and professional resources of resilience and agility in the healthcare workplace. *Stress and Health, 28*(1), 11–22. doi:10.1002/smi.1396

Plumb, C. (1995). *I'm no hero*. Mechanicsburg, PA: Tremendous Life Books.

Robertson, I. T., Cooper, C. L., Sarkar, M., & Curran, T. (2015). Resilience training in the workplace from 2003 to 2014: A systematic review. *Journal of Occupational and Organizational Psychology, 88*(3), 533–562. doi:10.1111/joop.12120

Rowland, J., & Baker, F. (2005). Resilience of cancer survivors across the lifespan. *Cancer, 101*(11, Suppl.), 2543–2548. doi:10.1002/cncr.21487

Schaufeli, W. B., Leiter, M. P., & Maslach, C. (2009). Burnout: 35 years of research and practice. *Career Development International, 14*(3), 204–220. doi:10.1108/13620430910966406

Schrecker, T. (2016). Globalization, austerity and health equity politics: Taming the inequality machine, and why it matters. *Critical Public Health, 26*(1), 4–13. doi:10.1080/09581596.2014.973019

Segal, J. (1986). *Winning life's toughest battles* (p. 130). New York, NY: McGraw-Hill.

Seligman, M. (1998). *Learned optimism*. New York, NY: Random House.

Selye, H. (1976). The stress concept. *Canadian Medical Association Journal, 115*(8), 718.

Siebert, A. (1996). *The survivor personality*. Berkley, CA: Perigee Books.

Slatyer, S., Craigie, M., Rees, C., Davis, S., Dolan, T., & Hegney, D. (2017). Nurse experience of participation in a mindfulness-based self-care and resiliency intervention. *Mindfulness, 9*, 1–8. doi:10.1007/s12671-017-0802-2

Smith, D. (2002). Functional salutogenic mechanisms of the brain. *Perspectives in Biology and Medicine, 45*(3), 319–328. doi:10.1353/pbm.2002.0058

Sroufe, L., Egeland, B., Carlson, E., & Collins, A. (2005). *The development of the person: The Minnesota study of risk and adaptation from birth to adulthood*. New York, NY: Guilford Press.

Stock, E. (2017). Exploring salutogenesis as a concept of health and wellbeing in nurses who thrive professionally. *British Journal of Nursing, 26*(4), 238–241. doi:10.12968/bjon.2017.26.4.238

Stockholm Resilience Centre. (2016). *Arctic resilience*. Stockholm: Author.

Suedfeld, P. (2005). Invulnerability, coping, salutogenesis, integration: Four phases of space psychology. *Aviation Space Environmental Medicine, 76*(6, Suppl. 1), B61–B66.

Sull, A., Harland, N., & Moore, A. (2015). Resilience of health-care workers in the UK: A cross-sectional survey. *Journal of Occupational Medicine and Toxicology, 10*(1), 20. doi:10.1186/s12995-015-0061-x

Tedeschi, R. G., & Calhoun, L. G. (2004). Posttraumatic growth: Conceptual foundations and empirical evidence. *Psychological Inquiry, 15*(1), 1–18. doi:10.1207/s15327965pli1501_01

Teixeira, M. E. (2008). Self-transcendence: A concept analysis for nursing praxis. *Holistic Nursing Practice, 22*(1), 25–31. doi:10.1097/01.HNP.0000306325.49332.ed

Walsh, F. (2015). *Strengthening family resilience*. New York, NY: Guilford Publications.

Werner, E., & Smith, R. (1982). *Vulnerable but invincible: A longitudinal study of resilient children and youth*. New York, NY: McGraw-Hill.

Wiesel, E. (1958). *Night*. New York, NY: Hill & Wang.

Wiesmann, U., & Hannich, H. J. (2010). A salutogenic analysis of healthy aging in active elderly persons. *Research on Aging, 32*(3), 349–371. doi:10.1177/0164027509356954

Windle, G., Bennett, K., & Noyes, J. (2011). A methodological review of resilience measurement scales. *Health and Quality of Life Outcomes, 9*, 8. doi:10.1186/1477-7525-9-8

# 2

# Historical Models of Resilience

Teddie Potter and Donna Lee Brien

## INTRODUCTION

One of the defining characteristics of modern life is an orientation toward the future. Nurses and nursing students are often very aware of the changes happening constantly in healthcare because of biotechnological discoveries and inventions. The future for health workers is awe-inspiring. As all workers, and all people more generally within society, need to contemplate the future and how it may change daily life, there is a formal interdisciplinary field called Future Studies or Futurology, which works to predict future trends and events (Bell, 2003). With change occurring at an unprecedented rate in almost all parts of life, in the future all aspects of existence, including work, will be very different from today in significant ways. Futurology proposes that it is, therefore, important that everyone in society—from governments, industry, businesses, professions, and organizations to single individuals— think about the future effects and ramifications of these changes, in order to make the best decisions now and face the future with a sense of optimism. As Futurology recognizes, however, purely forward-focused thinking not only diminishes conceptions of the value of the past, but can also limit the potential to understand both the present and the future. This chapter hones in on the notion that understanding the past can help nurses think more critically about both the present realities of, and future directions in, nursing and healthcare. We argue that this critical thinking is a life resource for making sense of challenging issues and wicked problems. It is, we believe, a resilience strategy—invaluable for nurses themselves, but also a strategy to encourage patients to consider. Thinking about the past illuminates the directions one wants to take in the future.

*Understanding the past can help nurses think more critically about both the present realities of, and future directions in, nursing and healthcare.*

In 1840, French historian and diplomat Alexis de Tocqueville wrote that, "When the past no longer illuminates the future, the spirit walks in darkness" (Project Gutenberg, 2013, n.p.), and many have paraphrased these thoughts about why a knowledge of the past is important. Peter N. Sterns (1998), the founding editor of the *Journal of Social History*, outlined a number of reasons why knowing about one's own history is important. He explains that history helps us understand not only "people and societies" (p. 2), but also "change and how the society we live in came to be" (p. 2). Additionally, Sterns also writes about how an understanding of history promotes the development of both "moral understanding" (p. 4) and a sense of one's identity, as well as making good citizens who contribute to society. Sterns also writes how a knowledge of history is useful in the working world—helping people think clearly and enhancing their abilities to adapt and be flexible (p. 8). More recently, Penelope Corfield has proposed that people are "living histories," the sum of all the legacies of the past (Corfield, 2008, n.p.). This recognizes that each individual inhabits a society whose languages, cultures, behaviors, and social norms have evolved over time.

Having an understanding about the past also has benefits beyond the level of the individual. In 2014, for instance, a report to the UK government formally outlined the positive—and essential—contribution a knowledge of the past makes to policy making (Haddon,

Devanny, Forsdick, & Thompson, 2014). In this, being aware of history was useful not just in terms of trying to not repeat the mistakes of the past and identifying useful models for contemporary decision-making, but also in helping to deal with change. This is because having historical knowledge enabled those with it to "challenge existing paradigms and identify major paradigm shifts" (Haddon et al., 2014, p. 2). Earlier work has recognized the importance of historical perspective for informed government (Neustadt & May, 1988) while recent research continues to stress the importance of a knowledge of history in a range of disciplines as diverse as business and marketing (Belasco & Scranton, 2014), teaching (Goldstein, 2014), and law (Ho, 2018).

Nursing has a rich and multilayered history as both a practice and a profession. A national study of nursing education (in Australia) found, however, that this history is neglected within the undergraduate nursing and midwifery curricula. This lack is, moreover, undermining students' ability to develop a strong professional nursing identity, and who are, instead

> a generation of professional orphans—unaware of who they are and where they've come from, unaware of reasons underlying cultural practices within the profession, lacking in vision for the future, insecure about their capacity to contribute to future directions, and not feeling part of something bigger and more enduring. (Madsen, McAllister, Godden, Greenhill, & Reed, 2009, p. 9)

The importance of teaching nursing history has also been echoed in studies in the United States (Alpers, Jarrell, & Wotring, 2011; American Association for the History of Nursing, 2001). When nursing history is taught, or discussed in nursing programs, it tends to focus on such famed and iconic figures such as Florence Nightingale, setting such heroic individuals and their actions apart from the "ordinary" nurses who provide day-to-day care today (MacDonald, De Zylva, McAllister, & Brien, 2018). A careful consideration of the autobiographies of some historic nursing leaders reveals, however, that—in many ways—these nurses were in fact also quite ordinary individuals. They chose, however, to act in extraordinary ways when confronted with challenges, and this is why their life stories are important to note.

There are many inspirational people in nursing's past; some of them are familiar to nurses all over the world, whereas others are well known only to a few. Some were formally trained as nurses, while others cared for patients before modern schools of nursing were opened. In very unique ways, they each chose to challenge the status quo by leading change and displayed great resilience in doing so. According to dictionary definitions, being resilient means being able to "withstand shock without permanent deformation or rupture" (Merriam-Webster, 2018, n.p.). In other words, to be able to bend without breaking. Many of the people considered to be the nursing profession's (heroic) ancestors were ordinary nurses, but nurses who responded to the challenges they faced with considerable resilience. Not only did they bend without breaking—which can be read as a somewhat passive reaction to stress—they also proactively turned their personal resilience into action and this had an effect on others and the profession of nursing.

For over 30 years, Kouzes and Posner have conducted research on the qualities of effective leaders. They have observed that, "All leaders *challenge the process*. Leaders are pioneers—people who are willing to step out into the unknown. They search for opportunities to innovate, grow, and improve" (2007, p. 17). The nurses discussed in the following all proactively faced and confronted challenging situations with resilience and, in doing so, led a positive transformation for either, or both, their patients and the nursing profession. Although they are heroes of nursing, it is their resilience and what this enabled them to do, that is of interest in this discussion.

## FLORENCE NIGHTINGALE (1820–1910)

Florence Nightingale was from a well-to-do British family (Figure 2.1). Even at an early age, she announced to her family that she had a Christian calling to become a nurse. Her parents were outraged because nursing was not, at that time, a career for respectable women, but she persevered in what became her vocation. She also had to overcome the restrictions of a healthcare system where medicine was valued far more than the kind of care, which could be, and was, offered by nurses. In her classic work, *Notes on Nursing: What It Is and What It*

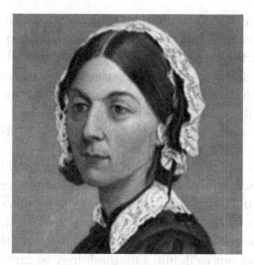

**Figure 2.1** Florence Nightingale, 1873.

*Is Not* (1860/1969), Nightingale acknowledged: "So deep-rooted and universal is the conviction that to give medicine is to be doing something, rather everything; to give air, warmth, cleanliness, etc., is to do nothing" (p. 9). Instead of feeling diminished or broken by the restrictive professional hierarchies she experienced in the healthcare system, Florence took action, using her keen knowledge of statistics and the scientific method in order to advance nursing as a unique profession.

It can be seen that Nightingale met the challenges of her time with considerable resilience. Despite resistance, she championed nurses' role in observing and acting on early indications of changes in health status. She wrote that such observation was critical:

> In all diseases it is important, but in diseases that do not run a distinct and fixed course, it is not only important, it is essential that the facts the nurse alone can observe should be accurately observed, and accurately reported. (p. 122)

Nightingale also challenged the hierarchical thinking of the day. Questioning the medical thinking that was then current, she courageously claimed that nature, not human intervention, actually performed the healing:

Surgery removes the bullet out of the limb, which is an obstruction to cure, but nature heals the wound. So it is with medicine; the function of an organ becomes obstructed; medicine, so far as we know, assists nature to remove the obstruction, but does nothing more. And what nursing has to do in either case is to put the patient in the best condition for nature to act upon him. (Nightingale, 1860/1969, p. 133)

During the Crimean War, Nightingale put many of her ideas into action in the Scutari Barracks in Istanbul. Her attentive observation of wounded soldiers at night earned her the moniker, "The Lady with the Lamp." Nightingale understood that fresh air, cleanliness, light, warmth, food, and attention to noise are the essence of healing and set out to define a methodology of care according to her beliefs (Nightingale, 1860/1969). She insisted that nurses be given uniforms, training, and instructions on how to improve the sanitation and the personal care of patients. Most of her efforts were not supported by the mainstream medical system of her day, but Nightingale was resilient in maintaining her course and staying true to her beliefs. As a result, she implemented changes that saved lives and forever altered the practice of nursing as well as the principles of healthcare more generally. She also brought about a profound change in how nursing as a profession is seen by the world. Although her legacy has been debated (Gill & Gill, 2005; Royle, 2000), her resilience is not to be challenged, and much can be learned from how she took an active stand against what she perceived as lacks and limitations in the system as it then existed, and how the idea of the professionalization of nursing remained at the fore of her thinking.

## MARY SEACOLE (1805–1881)

Mary Seacole was born in Kingston, Jamaica (Figure 2.2). Her father was Scottish and her mother was Jamaican. Mary learned about herbal remedies and folk medicine from her mother who ran a boarding house for disabled soldiers. She overcame several traumas while still young. In the 1830s, she married a merchant, but he was sickly and his business did not prosper. In the 1840s, her family's boarding house burned down; then, her mother died, followed by her husband.

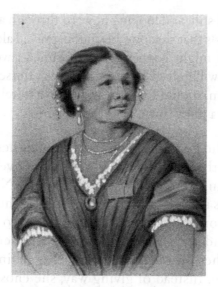

**Figure 2.2** Mary Seacole (drawing).

Mary took to her bed in grief, but soon composed herself, not only rejoining the world, but also taking over her mother's business and expanding her own nursing skills by traveling through the British colonies. Here she encountered and managed several epidemics of cholera and yellow fever.

Learning about the Crimean war and the high number of British fatalities, Seacole travelled to Britain to volunteer in the war effort. However, perhaps because of prejudice, she was refused and, when Nightingale successfully convinced the army to allow a group of female nurses to go to the Crimea, Mary was not among those selected. In her autobiography, Seacole (1857/2005) wrote of her awareness of why she had been rejected, and how painful this was:

> Did these ladies shrink from accepting aid because my blood flowed beneath a somewhat duskier skin than theirs? Tears streamed down my foolish cheeks, as I stood in the fast thinning streets; tears of grief that any should doubt my motives—that heaven should deny my opportunity that I sought. (pp. 73–74)

She did not, however, allow this hurdle to stop her, or let herself get distracted by self-pity. Instead, she responded creatively to this barrier in her path:

Then I stood still, and looking upward through and through the dark clouds that shadowed London, prayed aloud for help . . . Let what might happen, to the Crimea I would go . . . I would have willingly given my services as a nurse; but as they declined them, should I not go and open a hotel for invalids in the Crimea in my own way? (pp. 73–74)

And so she did go to the Crimea, but under her own auspices. She also made the most of this situation, actively seeking out ways of providing care and assistance. While Nightingale and the other nurses stayed within the confines of the army hospital in which they worked, Seacole ventured out onto the battlefield, selling goods and services. As well as moving her to action, her resilience kept her own identity from being defined and limited by someone else. Instead of giving way, she chose to rise above the societal prejudice she faced to follow her calling. She did not break and instead of reacting negatively, she took positively focused action for the benefit of many. Seacole wrote, "I love to be of service . . . And wherever the need arises—on whatever distant shore—I ask no greater or higher privilege than to minister to it" (1857/2005, p. 31).

> *These figures are role models for nursing because they were able to: (a) bend without breaking; and (b) turn their personal resilience into action.*

## WALT WHITMAN (1819–1892)

Women were not the only nurses who faced barriers in the 19th-century healthcare system because of their gender. Walt Whitman may be widely recognized as one of America's greatest poets, but few may know that he, too, overcame considerable societal prejudice to deliver nursing care to those in need; in his case, during the American Civil War (Figure 2.3). Of this work, he wrote:

I supply often to some of these dear suffering boys in my presence and magnetism that which doctors nor medicines nor skills nor any routine assistance can give . . . I can testify

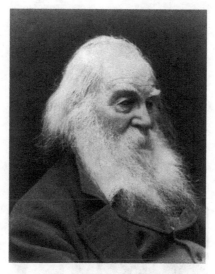

**Figure 2.3** Walt Whitman as an older man.
*Source:* George C. Cox, Library of Congress, USA, digital ID cph.3b20763.

that friendship has literally cured a fever, and the medicine of daily affection, a bad wound. (cited in Morris, 2000, p. 6)

This radical (for the time) attention to the holistic human and psychological needs of wounded and dying soldiers were precursors to hospice nursing today. Whitman saw a need, took action, and used his empathy to provide relationship-based care under the direst of conditions. Instead of being limited by the gender stereotypes of his day, Whitman stepped in and was resilient in the face of considerable resistance and, as a result, he was able to deliver this much-needed care.

## SISTER ELIZABETH KENNY (1880–1952)

Elizabeth Kenny dedicated herself to learning enough from others that she was able to become a district nurse in rural Australia (Figure 2.4). She volunteered as a nurse during World War I and, for her service, the Australian Army Nurse Corps awarded her the rank of "Sister" which is equivalent to that of first Lieutenant.

After the war, Kenny returned to Queensland and, during a 1930s outbreak of what is commonly known today as polio, developed an

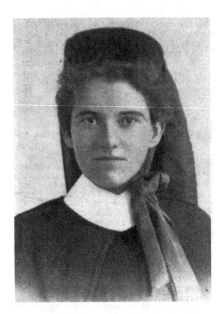

**Figure 2.4** Sister Elizabeth Kenny, photographed as she went to nurse in England during World War I, Brisbane, 1915.

*Source:* John Oxley Library, State Library of Queensland.

unconventional treatment for children suffering with acute polio-myelitis. Established medical treatment of the day for this disease required immobilization of the limbs with plaster casts or braces; however, Kenny advocated hot packs and passive exercises. Children who were treated with Kenny's method experienced significantly fewer polio-related disabilities than children who underwent the conventional medical treatment. Despite this successful treatment—and in part because this challenged current medical thinking—Kenny and her what were then seen as radical treatments were not well received by the medical establishment. While understanding the necessity for evidence-based practice, Kenny was saddened by the medical conservatism that was limiting innovation:

> I can understand how necessary it may be that new methods should be examined critically and that all the evidence must be carefully weighed before approval can be given. But I have also wondered how many promising discoveries have been consigned to oblivion without being given an opportunity to prove their worth. (Kenny & Ostenso, 1943, p. 2)

She also wrote of how astounded she was at the resistance she faced: "I was wholly unprepared for the extraordinary attitude of the medical world in its readiness to condemn anything that smacked of reform or that ran contrary to approved methods of practice" (quoted in Kenny & Ostenso, 1943, p. 2).

Despite this conservatism and lack of understanding of her methods, Sister Elizabeth Kenny did not give up. Instead she continued to believe in herself and what she had discovered, took action, and led a major change in medical practice. She achieved this, in part, by looking outside of her current environment for support. Leaving Australia, she traveled to the well-regarded Mayo Clinic in Minnesota in the United States where physicians were impressed with her results. Eventually, as a result of her perseverance and persistence in the face of doubt, Kenny Treatments Centers opened all around Australia and thousands of children and adults affected by polio learned to walk again.

> *Sometimes resilience involves taking action that goes against mainstream thinking in order to respond to moral imperatives.*

## LEARNING FROM THESE RESILIENT NURSES

These nurses—Nightingale, Seacole, Whitman, and Kenny—all exemplify the qualities of resilient nursing. They not only endured hostility, doubt, ignorance and prejudice, they also bent in the face of the resistance they faced. They were not broken and, to the contrary, each courageously took action to advance,provide, and bring about better standards of care and treatment to patients, and to advance the profession of nursing. These nurses not only had ideas to share with nursing and society, but they also took a stand when faced with prejudice and resistance to their actions and ideas, and ensured that their ideas and the changes that resulted were implemented. For these reasons, they can be seen to be part of the pantheon of nursing's heroes. It is important, however, to recognize that one does not have to directly experience such extremes of adversity in order to display such resilience. All nurses will encounter challenges at various points during their careers and should be ready to meet this with a resilient attitude.

These four nurses' leadership has been an important theme of this chapter. Posner and Kouzes list five characteristics of effective leaders: challenging the process; inspiring a shared vision; enabling others to act; modeling the way; and encouraging the heart (2017). In each case, these nurses' resilience enabled them to meet the challenges and resistance they faced and assume a leadership position in a situation that needed changing. These individuals exemplify the importance of action, *as well as* words, in being an effective and influential person. In different ways, each of these historical nursing figures showed leadership in order to bring about not just good practice, but—by bringing others along with them—to encourage enduring positive change in nursing and society. Chapter 4, The Resilience Standpoint in Nursing, discusses how these qualities of being proactive, of seeking to look to the welfare of nurses and their profession as well as of patients, and of considering the psychological and social ramifications of healthcare situations rather than the purely physical aspects of care, contribute to what can be called "the resilient standpoint."

## CONCLUSION

These stories illustrate the value of continuing to look back to the past to find stories of resilience-in-action in nursing history, in order to locate a source of inspiration for the present and guide confident and brave future actions. Much nursing history, as well as the biographies of resilient nurses, remains to be researched and written, and there is much work to be done to inspire others in the profession to engage with this history. Yet learning about, and from, the past has many benefits, including helping individuals to feel that they are not isolated, but part of a group that has a long history, and providing symbols of endurance and strength to emulate. Nursing history also reveals that some of the most innovative solutions in healthcare have come about when otherwise "ordinary" nurses resisted feeling helpless, claimed their power, moved beyond the dictates of the status quo, and innovated in order to bring about change. Today, every nurse has within his or her power the opportunity to not only respond to the challenges faced with resilience, but also to inspire and empower future nursing practice.

## LEARNING ACTIVITIES

1. Visit the Florence Nightingale Museum on the web, located at http://www.florence-nightingale.co.uk/index.php, to learn more about this inspirational leader and her contribution to the nursing profession.
2. Revisit Posner and Kouzes's (2017) characteristics of effective leaders:
   - Challenging the process
   - Inspiring a shared vision
   - Enabling others to act
   - Modeling the way
   - Encouraging the heart
3. What do you think "encouraging the heart" means? Think of someone from your life that you would consider being a good leader. How do they exemplify these characteristics?
4. For discussion: Think about the leadership qualities you might possess.
   - Are there some similarities you share with these historic nursing leaders?
   - Can you think of times when you conducted yourself in a manner similar to the way these leaders did?

## REFERENCES

Alpers, R. R., Jarrell, K., & Wotring, R. (2011). The importance of nursing history: A method of inclusion. *Teaching and Learning in Nursing*, 6(4), 190–191. doi:10.1016/j.teln.2011.08.001

American Association for the History of Nursing. (2001). Position paper: Nursing history in the curriculum: Preparing nurses for the 21st century. Retrieved from https://www.aahn.org/position-paper-on-history-in-curriculum

Belasco, W., & Scranton, P. (2014). *Food nations: Selling taste in consumer societies*. New York, NY: Routledge.

Bell, W. (2003). *Foundations of futures studies: Human science for a new era* (Rev. ed.). New Brunswick, NJ: Transaction Publishers.

Corfield, P. J. (2008). All people are living histories—Which is why history matters. *Making History*. Retrieved from http://www.history.ac.uk/makinghistory/resources/articles/why_history_matters.html

de Tocqueville, A. (1840). Democracy in America (Vol II, Ch. VIII. Henry Reeve, Trans.). Retrieved from Project Gutenberg (2013). https://www.gutenberg.org/files/816/816-h/816-h.htm#link2HCH0008

Gill, C. J., & Gill, G. C. (2005). Nightingale in Scutari: Her legacy reexamined. *Clinical Infectious Diseases, 40*(12), 1799–1805. doi:10.1086/430380

Goldstein, D. (2014). *The teacher wars: A history of America's most embattled profession*. New York, NY: Doubleday.

Haddon, C., Devanny, J., Forsdick, C., & Thompson, A. (2014). *What is the value of history in policymaking?* London, UK: Arts and Humanities Research Council and Institute for Government.

Ho, T. (2018). *The uses of history in determining what the law ought to be*. Doctoral thesis, University of Southern Queensland, Australia.

Kenny, E., & Ostenso, M. (1943). *And they shall walk*. New York, NY: Arno Press.

Kouzes, J. M., & Posner, B. Z. (2007). *The leadership challenge* (4th ed.). San Francisco, CA: Jossey-Bass.

MacDonald, K., De Zylva, J., McAllister, M., & Brien, D. L. (2018). Heroism and nursing: A thematic review of the literature. *Nurse Education Today, 68*, 134–140. doi:10.1016/j.nedt.2018.06.004

Madsen, W., McAllister, M., Godden, J., Greenhill, J., & Reed, R. (2009). Nursing's orphans: How the system of nursing education in Australia is undermining professional identity. *Contemporary Nurse, 32*(1–2), 9–18. doi:10.5172/conu.32.1-2.9

Merriam-Webster. (2018). Online dictionary: Resilient. Retrieved from https://www.merriam-webster.com/dictionary/resilient

Morris, R. (2000). *The better angel: Walt Whitman in the civil war*. Oxford, UK: Oxford University Press.

Neustadt, R. E., & May, E. R. (1988). *Thinking in time: The uses of history for decision makers*. New York, NY: Simon & Schuster.

Nightingale, F. (1969). *Notes on nursing: What it is and what it is not*. New York, NY: Dover Books on Biology. (Original work published 1860)

Posner, B. Z., & Kouzes, J. M. (2017). 5 practices of exemplary leadership. Retrieved from https://www.success.com/article/5-practices-of-exemplary-leadership

Royle, T. (2000). *Crimea: The great Crimean War, 1854–1856*. New York, NY: Saint Martin's Press.

Seacole, M. (2005). *Wonderful adventures of Mrs. Seacole in many lands*. New York, NY: Penguin Books. (Original work published 1857)

Sterns, P. N. (1998). Why study history? American Historical Association. Retrieved from https://www.historians.org/about-aha-and-membership/aha-history-and-archives/historical-archives/why-study-history-(1998)

# 3

# The "Wicked" Global Problems Facing Nursing

Ben Hannigan and Margaret McAllister

## INTRODUCTION

Nursing work is demanding. This is so across the full range of roles nurses fulfill. These roles include face-to-face clinical work with individuals, organizing nurses and others' work so that patients' journeys through health services are as seamless as possible, managing teams whose members share collective responsibilities for care provision, educating future nurses, and generating an evidence base through research. Nurses face pressure whether they work in hospitals, primary healthcare clinics, or in the homes of patients living in the community, and whether they are employed in public health roles, private businesses, or universities.

Yet opportunities to step away from the day-to-day rigors of work to reflect on what it is that makes nursing demanding are rare. This chapter offers an opportunity of this type. It provides an overview of some of the social, economic, political, organizational, technological, and professional challenges that nurses face. As we will demonstrate, many of these challenges are of the "wicked" variety, described as such because they are not easy to resolve and tend to keep recurring, and/or are endemic in certain contexts.

The intention of this chapter is that the analysis presented, and the practical activities offered, will interest, and be of use to, nurses at all levels of experience and seniority. This includes those approaching initial qualification, those who are newly registered or licensed, and those who occupy advanced clinical, managerial, or other roles. This overview will not (and cannot) be exhaustive, because the territory to be covered is vast. However, by the end of this chapter it is hoped that readers will have an understanding of some of the sources of pressure nurses face that place such a premium on nurses being resilient.

*Wicked problems in healthcare are those health issues that are entrenched within certain groups. They often have multiple or complex causes or solutions that are incomplete or inadequately implemented, and thus the problem persists and contributes to health inequities, disability, and ongoing suffering.*

## SOCIAL, ECONOMIC, AND POLITICAL CHALLENGES

In countries like Australia, the United States, and the UK, decades of economic development have delivered the benefits of high levels of national income and the creation of evolved health and social care systems. As a result, people are living longer and managing, rather than dying from, affliction and disease. The World Health Organization (WHO) publishes comprehensive, population-level, health-related data online (WHO, 2018). This provides important demographic and health expenditure information from around the world. Table 3.1 summarizes some key facts and figures. Forecasters looking ahead to the year 2030 project that life expectancy at birth in high-income countries will continue to increase, heading in some parts of the world toward almost 90 years of age for women and substantially over 80 years of age for men (Kontis et al., 2017). This is a remarkable achievement and is unparalleled in human history.

However, as populations around the world have aged, the prevalence of chronic health conditions also has grown. In industrialized nations almost half of the burden of disease is attributable to disorders experienced by those aged 60 years or over (Prince et al., 2015). Cardiovascular diseases, cancers, musculoskeletal diseases, mental and

Table 3.1 Population Level Data: Australia, the United States, and the UK

| | Total Population[1] | Life Expectancy at Birth (Male/Female)[1] | Total Expenditure on Health as % of Gross Domestic Product[2] |
|---|---|---|---|
| Australia | 23,969,000 | 81/85 | 9.4 |
| United States of America | 321,774,000 | 77/82 | 17.1 |
| United Kingdom | 64,716,000 | 79/83 | 9.1 |

[1]2015
[2]2014

Source: Data extracted from http://www.who.int/countries.

neurologic disorders, and chronic respiratory diseases all feature highly. As Prince et al. (2015, p. 549) put it, "The epidemiological transition from the age of pestilence and famine to the age of degenerative and man-made diseases is near complete in most high-income countries." This has important implications on health policy and practice and, therefore, the work of nurses. Public health initiatives to promote well-being and prevent disease across this extended life span have become of growing importance, as have initiatives and programs to support people to live well into old age with long-term disease and disability.

Dementia is an instructive example. Perhaps more than any other disease, dementia most obviously reflects aging populations. With one new case of dementia around the world every 7 seconds, dementia is most prevalent in industrialized countries, but the number of people affected is projected to increase at an accelerating rate in developing nations (Ferri et al., 2005). The total estimated worldwide costs of dementia in 2015 were US $818 billion, an increase of 35% over just 5 years (Wimo et al., 2017). It has also been estimated that the total cost of dementia exceeds the costs of cancer, stroke, and coronary heart disease combined (Luengo-Fernandez, Leal, & Gray, 2015). This underscores the vital importance of population-level as well as individual-level action, including interventions to address risk factors along with those to slow the course of the disease and to enable people to live independently for as long as possible.

With countries adjusting to meet the challenges of long-term conditions such as dementia, interest has grown in comparing and contrasting the different approaches taken by different governments and the various outcomes for patients resulting from these approaches. Descriptive information in this area is published by The Commonwealth Fund, which in 2017 produced its most recent comparison of international healthcare systems (Mossialos, Djordjevic, Osborn, & Sarnak, 2017). As this document reveals, health systems vary across a number of dimensions. These include:

- The proportion of national income devoted to healthcare
- The role played by the state in directly funding and/or providing services along with the corresponding part played by private organizations and insurers
- The types and numbers of health professionals educated and employed
- The numbers and availability of hospital beds
- Measures taken to promote integration and coordination across sectors
- Advances in the use of new technologies
- Measures taken to promote quality and safety

In Australia, government responsibilities for healthcare are located at three levels (federal, state and territory, and local) and universal coverage is provided through Medicare, a public health insurance program (Glover, 2017), which was instituted in 1984. In the United States, major extensions to healthcare coverage took place with the passing of the Patient Protection and Affordable Care Act (2010; known as "Obamacare"), which shares responsibility for funding healthcare among the government, employers, and individuals (The Commonwealth Fund, 2017). At the time of writing this chapter, the Affordable Care Act has faced significant challenge from the new U.S. administration under President Trump but has not been replaced. In the UK, responsibility for healthcare is devolved to elected governments across the four countries (England, Wales, Scotland, and Northern Ireland), but since the 1940s the National Health Service (NHS) has ensured that care is universally provided, with funding provided through general taxation (Thorlby & Arora, 2017).

Common across all these and other systems, irrespective of their organizational and funding differences, is the pressure to do more with less in the context of growing, and longer-lived, populations and ever-closer scrutiny of how resources are used. This scrutiny has become more pronounced following the global economic crash of 2008, which challenged many governments to sustain their health system funding (Quaglio, Karapiperis, Van Woensel, Arnold, & McDaid, 2013). In the wake of the economic crisis, many administrations around the world elected to pursue austerity policies, reducing public expenditure. However, when governments reduce expenditure, this has social consequences and there tends to be more unemployment, homelessness, food insecurity, rising levels of mental ill-health, cuts to social care and associated rises in mortality among older people (Stuckler, Reeves, Loopstra, Karanikolos, & McKee, 2017).

It is in this context that debates are often aired over what type of health system works best. The Commonwealth Fund produces regular performance reports, its most recent publication comparing health systems in 11 industrialized countries on 72 indicators spread across five domains (care process, access, administrative efficiency, equity, and healthcare outcomes; Schneider, Sarnak, Squires, Shah, & Doty, 2017). In this, the UK is top overall, with Australia second and the United States in last place, despite devoting far greater resources to healthcare than other advanced nations.

## ORGANIZATIONAL CHALLENGES: HEALTH AS A COMPLEX SYSTEM

While important differences exist in the politics and economics of health in different parts of the world, all health services can be thought of as examples of complex systems (Braithwaite et al., 2017; Plsek & Greenhalgh, 2001). A common feature of advanced, evolved health systems is that no single body has authority or responsibility to fulfill all the tasks that are required in each system. Modern systems are full of interacting parts, including commissioners, insurers, provider organizations, and professionals. Within these systems there are hierarchies and, as a result, lines of communication (e.g., between national-level policymakers, local managers, and frontline practitioners) are not always as clear as they might be. Systems also co-exist. For example, interfaces exist between primary healthcare and hospital-based systems, and between health systems and those centered on the provision of social care. There should be porous boundaries between systems so that interaction, communication, and sharing of ideas and resources can take place. Often, however, systems can become rigid and dysfunctional, and lines of communication, understanding, and efficiency are disturbed and ineffective.

The mental health field offers an excellent case example of this (Ellis, Churruca, & Braithwaite, 2017). Mental health systems have a history that stretches back to the era of the asylums of the 19th century and later (Hannigan & Allen, 2006). As these hospitals were built, opportunities emerged for new occupational groups to take their place within them, including psychiatrists and nurses. As the hospital era yielded to an era of community care in the years following the end of the Second World War, further opportunities arose for nurses, social workers, and others to expand their work caring for people with mental health difficulties who were increasingly living in their own homes rather than in institutions. Over time, an intricate division of labor has emerged, but at the same time, roles and responsibilities have sometimes become blurred (Hannigan & Allen, 2011). For example, both nurses and occupational therapists explore and theorize about clients' activities of daily living. In another example, nurse practitioners and medical practitioners are involved in prescribing medications and thus develop expertise in pharmacology. For an individual using mental health services, the range of organizations and professionals with parts to play in their care can seem thoroughly bewildering. In complex healthcare systems, like those found in Australia, the United States, and the UK, it is also usual for patients to move across multiple service interfaces during their journeys. Interfaces exist between primary healthcare teams and specialist services, between community teams and hospitals, and between different parts of either the hospital or community parts of the system. When crossing jurisdictions, laws are not always in place to enable sharing of information. Sometimes, information can be lost and care discontinuities ensue, with negative implications for the quality of care and advice provided and, as a result, patient safety. This emphasizes the need for coordination of care, by which the patient is brought to the system and the system is brought to the person (Hannigan & Allen, 2013).

High-profile cases exist of discontinuities of care leading to people becoming lost to health and social care systems, sometimes with tragic consequences. In the UK, for instance, the case of

Christopher Clunis is often cited as an example, not least because of the longer-term impact on services that it had. Clunis had severe · paranoid schizophrenia, and frequently admitted to hearing voices telling him to kill someone, and in 1992 stabbed a stranger at a London underground station. In the subsequent inquiry into this killing, it was found that Clunis had been moved between different services, and information had not always been passed on from one care coordinator to another each time he moved (Ritchie, Dick, & Lingham, 1994). Healthcare practitioners were either worried that his history of severe mental instability would deter other health workers from accepting him or did not want to bias his care and delay referrals. However, not knowing proved to be more dangerous and Clunis was not provided with the intensive care needed to relieve his symptoms and provide for the safety of him and the community. Policy and practice for care coordination have developed considerably since that time, but the fact that multiple professionals (and others) are still required to work together in the care of individuals with multiple needs continues to present both an organizational challenge—and, for some, a personal challenge.

## THE CHALLENGE OF "WICKED" PROBLEMS

Not all problems are easy to solve. Some problems even have an appearance of intractability which challenges attempts to precisely define what "the problem" actually is. "Wicked problems," as these problems are sometimes called (Rittel & Webber, 1973), are particularly hard to resolve and they are also exactly the type of problem which are most likely to vex governments. Problems of this type are often deeply intertwined with others, so that one problem turns out to be connected to another of equal magnitude. Many of the challenges facing nurses and other healthcare practitioners are of this type (Hannigan & Coffey, 2011). An example is that of health inequalities (Blackman et al., 2006). It is well-known that, within single nations, positive health and wellbeing is not enjoyed equally by all members of the population. In Australia, for example, there are strong inequalities between the health status and determinants of health amongst indigenous and non-indigenous Australians, and between low and high socioeconomic groups (Australian Institute of Health and Welfare, 2015). A recent Australian Institute of Health and

Welfare report shows how, for instance, indigenous people experience higher rates of mental health problems, respiratory disease (amongst older age groups), cardiovascular disease, and diseases of the kidneys and other organs along with high rates of disability. Despite decades of interventions, this problem has not been solved.

*Significant gaps between indigenous and non-indigenous Australians remain. This is a wicked problem because it involves disadvantages in areas such as such as health, housing, education, and employment.*

There are also, however, outstanding examples of success and these are important to share so that stereotypes and pessimism can be transformed into a determination to collaborate with others or to at least try to resolve such issues. These successes also demonstrate how progress can be made to tackle even the most complex challenges. In Brisbane, Australia, for example, there is a vivid example of an innovative solution to such endemic problems. In this city, there is an Aboriginal and Torres Strait Islander-controlled health service that has been operating since the 1970s. The service is rightly proud of their successes. They have achieved the following:

- The doubling of patient visits to doctors between 2009 and 2011
- An increase of thousands of new patients
- Increased use of dental care
- The opening of two new clinics
- More jobs for indigenous people
- Higher levels of stability in diabetes, smoking rates, cholesterol and blood pressure (Korff, 2016).

At the broader social level, Wilkinson and Pickett (2010) explain the many ways in which inequality damages individuals and whole societies. They show how income differentials within countries are associated with a wide range of physical and mental health inequalities. They also demonstrate how income disparities are associated with other inequalities including literacy and numeracy, social mobility, and rates of homicide.

Therefore, tackling health inequalities means also tackling other (equally large) problems such as poverty, homelessness, and unemployment. Whilst there is much for health services and professionals to do to pursue this kind of "joined-up" action, much also has to be done by organizations and people in other, interconnected, sectors. Schools, colleges, and universities, private and public employers, local and national governments and others can all make a contribution but joining up these various contributions in a concerted fashion is exceptionally challenging.

*Tackling health inequalities means also tackling other problems such as poverty, homelessness, and unemployment, which is why nurses need to extend their biomedical skills to include psychosocial collaborative actions.*

## THE WORLD OF WORK: PROFESSIONS AND PRACTICES

The profession of nursing is not static but continues to evolve in response to wider social, political, economic, and technological change and to developments internally within the profession itself. One important evolution has been the emergence in many, but not all, countries of nursing as an independent profession complete with its own knowledge base, control over entry to its ranks and the authority to license its members and simultaneously award university-level degrees. The WHO now specifies global standards for the education of nurses, recognizing at the same time how the preparation of nurses has historically varied across the world (WHO, 2009). These standards are explicit in recommending nursing as a graduate-level profession, in which new entrants should be eligible for further, advanced, education reflecting the expansion of their roles. More recently, the WHO has recognized the contribution nurses make to health improvement and to the efficient and effective running of health systems (WHO, 2016).

However, despite global endorsements of this type, nursing remains a profession under threat. This is despite important research evidencing that more, and better educated, nurses are associated with better patient outcomes. Using discharge data for 422,730 surgical patients in 300 hospitals in nine European countries, along with survey data from 26,516 practicing nurses, a research project published in 2014 (Aiken et al., 2014) investigated the relationships between numbers of nurses, their qualifications, and outcomes for surgical patients. They found that patients in hospitals where 60% of nurses had undergraduate degrees and cared for an average of six patients had almost 30% lower mortality than patients in hospitals in which only 30% of nurses had bachelor's degrees and nurses cared for an average of eight patients. Healthy staffing levels, with care provided by graduate nurses is clearly, therefore, a route to preventing deaths. In the face of evidence of this type, however, nursing still suffers from outdated and stereotyped representation in the media and popular imagination (Darbyshire, 2010; Stanley, 2012). Nurses, unlike other health professional groups, are rarely consulted when policy and service change is mooted. Many find their everyday working conditions to be quite unlike what they imagined when they decided on nursing as a career, and baulk at the high levels of administration, poor team work and high levels of stress and burnout typically experienced in the workplace (Hanson & McAllister, 2017).

Changes in working practices, the emergence of novel roles and evolving new technologies are also exerting an impact on the work and experiences of nurses. Patients who were once cared for in hospital are now nursed at home, and work which was once done by one type of professional is now being done by others, or teams of carers. New knowledge, skills, and competencies need to be developed over the lifetime of a typical nursing career, which with the pushing back of retirement ages in many parts of the world, is becoming ever longer. Navigating the changing world of work is becoming increasingly demanding, and resilience is important in this context.

## CONCLUSION

Given the challenges outlined in this chapter, it is reasonable to ask: what type of nurse is best able to not only survive, but also to thrive, in contemporary health services? The answer is, the nurse who is resilient. This is the nurse possessing an awareness of changing population needs and of the implications of these changing needs for healthcare organization and practice. The resilient nurse has knowledge of the system within which they operate and is able to communicate effectively across interfaces and to coordinate services and care. This is an individual who also perceives the bigger picture and is able to place the patient in his or her social and economic context. The resilient nurse knows the importance of partnerships, and of partners and teams working together to tackle the causes as well as the consequences of poor health. They also know the value of education and are capable of articulating (and defending) the work of nurses and of challenging outmoded and damaging stereotypes. Individually, the resilient nurse is not only able to give support to, but also to receive support from, others.

## LEARNING ACTIVITIES

1. The opening section of this chapter traced the social and economic challenges facing health systems, and therefore nurses, in high-income countries. This activity invites you to put yourself in the shoes of a newly elected government minister with responsibility for healthcare in the country in which you live and work. Your task is to write an open letter, of not more than 300 words, outlining the challenges you face, your priorities for change, and the specific actions you plan to take in your first year in office. Discuss your letter with a peer, and if she or he would also write a letter of this type, and compare and contrast your thinking on this topic.

2. Identify a healthcare workplace with which you are familiar: this could be the area in which you currently practice, or in which you have had a recent clinical placement as a student. Next, select a patient or client of this service, and reflect on his or her journey into, through, and out of the system. Avoid using any real names or other identifiers, but consider the person's journey into, through and out of the service.
   - How many practitioners were involved, at what points, and how did they hand care over?
   - Did any confusions arise, on the part of the patient or amongst professionals?
   - Did the patient appreciate, or become puzzled by, the segmented care? Did they have any other reaction(s)?
   - Was information on the progress of the patient shared amongst the team, including with the person making the original referral?

- Was the patient (and their carers) asked about the effectiveness of this journey, and did they have any complaints or compliments?
- What might have helped improve the flow of work and the exchange of information?
- Overall, how effectively was this person's care coordinated?

3. This chapter suggests that some problems are intimately intertwined, which makes challenging them difficult. This does not mean that nurses (and others) should feel powerless, however, as the example from Brisbane demonstrates. The Australian Public Service Commission has published a document, *Tackling wicked problems*, which outlines principles and practical strategies for meeting the challenge (Australian Public Service Commission, 2007). In this, obesity is correctly described as an example of a wicked problem. Any solution to obesity is likely to involve changes to not only individual behavior but also to food production, sales and marketing practices, to school and workplace canteen procedures, in the organization of the working day, in the shape of the built environment, and in the availability and accessibility of sports and leisure facilities (Finegood, Merth, & Rutter, 2010). While nurses can obviously not achieve all this, they have a real opportunity in their day-to-day work to not only influence patient behavior, but also to lobby for wider change. Imagine yourself as the Lead Public Health Nurse for the organization in which you work. Your task is to produce recommendations for a strategy to reduce obesity in your territory, city or town. Things to consider include:
   - Who are your partners in this strategy (schools, colleges, local authorities, employers, etc.)?
   - What joined-up actions do you propose, and at what levels (e.g., targeting individual behavior, local food production and consumption, increasing uptake of sport and leisure activities)?
   - Specifically, what do you expect nurses to do in their everyday work, and in their different workplaces, to contribute to your strategy?

4. Imagine you are the Director of Nursing at your local hospital and are planning a major new recruitment drive. You need to

write a welcome piece to accompany your advertisements. What vision for nursing professionals will you try to convey, and how would you like to present your organization to potential new recruits? What do you need to write to express the idea that nurses are valued, supported in their personal development and involved in decision-making at all levels? Write a 200-word promotional flyer.

## REFERENCES

Aiken, L. H., Sloane, D. M., Bruyneel, L., Van den Heede, K., Griffiths, P., Busse, R., . . . for the RN4CAST consortium. (2014). Nurse staffing and education and hospital mortality in nine European countries: A retrospective observational study. *The Lancet, 383*(9931), 1824–1830. doi:10.1016/S0140-6736(13)62631-8

Australian Institute of Health and Welfare. (2015). *The health and welfare of Australia's Aboriginal and Torres Strait Islander peoples 2015*. Canberra: Author.

Australian Public Service Commission. (2007). *Tackling wicked problems: A public policy perspective*. Canberra: Australian Government.

Blackman, T., Elliott, E., Greene, A., Harrington, B., Hunter, D. J., Marks, L., . . . Williams, G. (2006). Performance assessment and wicked problems: The case of health inequalities. *Public Policy and Administration, 21*(2), 66–80. doi:10.1177/095207670602100206

Braithwaite, J., Churruca, K., Ellis, L. A., Long, J., Clay-Williams, R., Damen, N., . . . Ludlow, K. (2017). *Complexity science in healthcare: Aspirations, approaches, applications and accomplishments: A White Paper*. Sydney: Australian Institute for Health Innovation, Macquarie University.

Darbyshire, P. (2010). Heroines, hookers and harridans: Exploring popular images and representations of nurses and nursing. In J. Daly, S. Speedy, & D. Jackson (Eds.), *Contexts of nursing* (pp. 51–64). Chatswood, NSW: Elsevier.

Ellis, L. A., Churruca, K., & Braithwaite, J. (2017). Mental health services conceptualised as complex adaptive systems: What can be learned? *International Journal of Mental Health Systems, 11*, 43. doi:10.1186/s13033-017-0150-6

Ferri, C. P., Prince, M., Brayne, C., Brodaty, H., Fratiglioni, L., Ganguli, M., . . . Scazufca, M. (2005). Global prevalence of dementia: A Delphi consensus study. *The Lancet, 366*(9503), 2112–2117. doi:10.1016/S0140-6736(05)67889-0

Finegood, D. T., Merth, T. D. N., & Rutter, H. (2010). Implications of the Foresight obesity system map for solutions to childhood obesity. *Obesity, 18*(Suppl. 1), S13–S16. doi:10.1038/oby.2009.426

Glover, L. (2017). The Australian health care system. In E. Mossialos, A. Djordjevic, R. Osborn, & D. Sarnak (Eds.), *International profiles of health care systems*. New York, NY: The Commonwealth Fund.

Hannigan, B., & Allen, D. (2006). Complexity and change in the United Kingdom's system of mental health care. *Social Theory & Health, 4*(3), 244–263. doi:10.1057/palgrave.sth.8700073

Hannigan, B., & Allen, D. (2011). Giving a fig about roles: Policy, context and work in community mental health care. *Journal of Psychiatric and Mental Health Nursing, 18*(1), 1–8. doi:10.1111/j.1365-2850.2010.01631.x

Hannigan, B., & Allen, D. (2013). Complex caring trajectories in community mental health: Contingencies, divisions of labor and care coordination. *Community Mental Health Journal, 49*(4), 380–388. doi:10.1007/s10597-011-9467-9

Hannigan, B., & Coffey, M. (2011). Where the wicked problems are: The case of mental health. *Health Policy, 101*(3), 220–227. doi:10.1016/j.healthpol.2010.11.002

Hanson, J., & McAllister, M. (2017). Preparation for workplace adversity: Student narratives as a stimulus for learning. *Nurse Education in Practice, 25*, 89–95. doi:10.1016/j.nepr.2017.05.008

Kontis, V., Bennett, J. E., Mathers, C. D., Li, G., Foreman, K., & Ezzat, M. (2017). Future life expectancy in 35 industrialised countries: Projections with a Bayesian model ensemble. *The Lancet, 389*(10076), 1323–1335. doi:10.1016/S0140-6736(16)32381-9

Korff, J. (2016). Successful Aboriginal health services. *Creative Spirits.* Retrieved from https://www.creativespirits.info/aboriginalculture/health/successful-aboriginal-health-services#ixzz5B0yVLQss

Luengo-Fernandez, R., Leal, J., & Gray, A. (2015). UK research spend in 2008 and 2012: Comparing stroke, cancer, coronary heart disease and dementia. *BMJ Open, 5*(4), e006648. doi:10.1136/bmjopen-2014-006648

Mossialos, E., Djordjevic, A., Osborn, R., & Sarnak, D. (Eds.). (2017). *International profiles of health care systems.* New York, NY: The Commonwealth Fund.

Plsek, P. E., & Greenhalgh, T. (2001). The challenge of complexity in health care. *BMJ, 323*(7313), 625–628. doi:10.1136/bmj.323.7313.625

Prince, M. J., Wu, F., Guo, Y., Gutierrez Robledo, L. M., O'Donnell, M., Sullivan, R., & Yusuf, S. (2015). The burden of disease in older people and implications for health policy and practice. *The Lancet, 385*(9967), 549–562. doi:10.1016/S0140-6736(14)61347-7

Quaglio, G., Karapiperis, T., Van Woensel, E., Arnold, E., & McDaid, D. (2013). Austerity and health in Europe. *Health Policy, 113*(1–2), 13–19. doi:10.1016/j.healthpol.2013.09.005

Ritchie, J. H., Dick, D., & Lingham, R. (1994). *The report of the inquiry into the care and treatment of Christopher Clunis.* London, UK: HMSO.

Rittel, H. W. J., & Webber, M. W. (1973). Dilemmas in a general theory of planning. *Policy Sciences, 4*(2), 155–169. doi:10.1007/BF01405730

Schneider, E. C., Sarnak, D. O., Squires, D., Shah, A., & Doty, M. M. (2017). *Mirror, mirror 2017: International comparison reflects flaws and opportunities for better US health care.* New York, NY: The Commonwealth Fund.

Stanley, D. (2012). Celluloid devils: A research study of male nurses in feature films. *Journal of Advanced Nursing, 68*(11), 2526–2537. doi:10.1111/j.1365-2648.2012.05952.x

Stuckler, D., Reeves, A., Loopstra, R., Karanikolos, M., & McKee, M. (2017). Austerity and health: The impact in the UK and Europe. *European Journal of Public Health, 27*(Suppl. 4), 18–21. doi:10.1093/eurpub/ckx167

The Commonwealth Fund. (2017). The US health care system. In E. Mossialos, A. Djordjevic, R. Osborn, & D. Sarnak (Eds.), *International profiles of health care systems*. New York, NY: Author.

Thorlby, R., & Arora, S. (2017). The English health care system. In E. Mossialos, A. Djordjevic, R. Osborn, & D. Sarnak (Eds.), *International profiles of health care systems*. New York, NY: The Commonwealth Fund.

Wilkinson, R., & Pickett, K. (2010). *The spirit level: Why equality is better for everyone*. London, UK: Penguin.

Wimo, A., Guerchet, M., Ali, G. C., Wu, Y. T., Prina, M., Winblad, B., . . . Prince, M. (2017). The worldwide costs of dementia 2015 and comparisons with 2010. *Alzheimer's and Dementia, 13*(1), 1–7. doi:10.1016/j.jalz.2016.07.150

World Health Organization. (2009). *Global standards for the initial education of professional nurses and midwives*. Geneva, Switzerland: Author.

World Health Organization. (2016). *Global strategic directions for strengthening nursing and midwifery 2016-2020*. Geneva, Switzerland: Author.

World Health Organization (2018). Countries. Retrieved from http://www.who .int/countries

# 4

# The Resilience Standpoint in Nursing

Margaret McAllister and Donna Lee Brien

## INTRODUCTION

Taking a stand on something requires developing a clear set of beliefs and a point of view from which you will not veer. This means you have a standpoint. Standpoint theory comes from feminism, and the awareness that the main way to resolve the ongoing marginalization of women is to have a clear point of view about women's right to be heard and respected, *and* that these rights are repeatedly dismissed because of a tendency for "male-centric" ideas to dominate thinking and become commonplace (Harding, 2004). To maintain a feminist standpoint means that one puts women's rights at the center of thinking and acting. You stand up for women, and check for any anti-female biases and stigmatizing views before engaging in any interactions.

Given that resilience is so important for nursing, we thought it would be useful to develop a point of view about resilience and what it means, or could mean, for nursing.

A resilience standpoint can be characterized as follows:

1. Nurses form the basis of any healthcare system and understand that health is more than the absence of disease or illness.

Therefore, nurses must play a role in building resilience in clients and communities. To be an "illness-care" worker is insufficient because this mode of operation, despite being commonplace in healthcare systems, is reactive and only treatment oriented. Illness care does not proactively build wellness, and nurses should play a role in health promotion, illness prevention, and the generation of wellness and well-being.

2. Resilience has a double purpose for nursing. Understanding and operationalizing it is part of a nurse's toolkit when working with clients, but it is also something that can be directed inwardly toward the self and outwardly toward the profession. In this way, resilience strategies can be utilized *with and for* patients, as well as *with and for* nursing.

3. Resilience involves psychological as well as social strengthening. Even though most of the research into resilience has focused on, and emanated from, psychological science, there is much to be learned from cultural studies focusing on resilient communities and the actions small groups have taken to overcome obstacles, build a strong identity, and live healthy, peaceful, rewarding lives. To enact resilience strategies as a nurse therefore requires psychosocial competence and some perseverance. This is developed through education and training that focuses on skill development.

Developing and then maintaining such a standpoint toward resilience in nursing can be useful in forming the starting point for nursing actions with clients, and in the processes of developing resilient teams, organizations, and healthcare networks.

## COMMONPLACE VIEWS OF STRONG NURSES

Nurses are often portrayed as surmounting enormous challenges with courage and grace (Stanley, 2008). This is a flattering image for nurses, but it has become so commonplace that people have wrongly conflated the actions of heroic nurses who have achieved extraordinary things with the inherent traits that all nurses share. But not all nurses are born strong or endowed with the traits of resiliency. This chapter draws on the resilience standpoint to critique such descriptions and suggest a more sustainable way to imagine nurses and nursing.

Epic portrayals of nursing are common in images of nurses during wars, such as in the First World War, and other dramatic situations. In such representations, nurses are often imaged as acting heroically and coping with enormous difficulties efficiently and stoically. This strength is also commonly framed around personal and individual capabilities that are so recognizable as to be stereotypes—like nurses' caring nature (Kelly, Fealy, & Watson, 2012). The iconic figure in nursing history—that of Florence Nightingale—is a prominent and enduring example. She first became well known and admired as a public figure during the Crimean War in the 1850s when she established a hospital near the Front. This hospital did not just care for the wounded, but also improved hygiene conditions, and conducted research on morbidity and mortality rates. *The White Angel* (Diertele, 1936), a classic film about Nightingale and her work that can be still be accessed today in archives and various online sites, conjures up an image about nursing that resonates today—that nurses are (expected to be) strong, selfless individuals. Nightingale went on to establish a training system for nurses that was based around learning about care and the promotion of a work ethic of service, duty, and personal containment, as well as dignified comportment even in the face of horrifying injuries, fatigue, and grueling working conditions (Meyer & Bishop, 2007).

Contemporary nurses are expected to live up to this mythic ideal that they have an inherently caring nature, and need to be compliant workers, expectant of nothing except gratitude (Levett-Jones & Lathlean, 2009). In this schema, any personal satisfaction is meant to come from the quiet knowledge of how well the caring task they have performed has been achieved. This stereotype, and the so-called virtue script it generates and follows (Gordon & Nelson, 2006) contributes to a prevailing concept of resilience as a psychological trait (Tugade, Fredrickson, & Feldman Barrett, 2004) that assists the nurses in this achievement.

As we have seen in previous chapters, early psychological research considered the personal capacity for resilience (termed "resiliency") to involve four distinct features. Resiliency is, thus, a psychological capacity, while resilience is the more overarching term that encompasses psychological capacity as well as social and environmental factors, and that all contribute to the state of resilience. The first trait of resiliency is hardiness. "Stress hardy" individuals understand stress as a challenge and an opportunity for growth rather than a problem (Kobasa, 1979). An example of such a trait is seen in Edith Cavell, the First World War nurse who remained brave and stoic to the end. After having nursed soldiers on both sides of the conflict and, as a result, having been accused by the German military of treason, she was executed by firing squad (Forrester, 2016). Her stoicism is taken to be bravery in performing the ultimate act of care, sacrificing herself for helping others.

Holding an internal locus of control is another trait of resiliency. In enacting self-control, the individuals believe themselves to share responsibility in both a problem and its management (Rotter, 1966). Walt Whitman illustrates this attribute. At the start of the American Civil War, Whitman was a journalist who visited wounded patients and asked them to tell him their stories in order to inform the public about what was occurring during the fighting. After realizing that he could do more, and that he had a responsibility to act, he changed his focus to provide direct nursing care to these wounded men, care that he continued to perform for several years.

A third feature of resiliency is the ability to not be flattened by—and to be able to bounce back from—adversity (Tugade & Frederickson, 2004). When they do fall, individuals who display this trait do not break but instead rebound. Mary Seacole is a clear example of someone displaying this kind of resiliency. As an experienced healer, who had tended to soldiers for many years in her homeland of Jamaica, she responded to Nightingale's call for nurses to join her in the Crimea. When she was rejected, Seacole was disappointed but not deterred. Instead, she self-funded her own travel to the war zone and set up her own nursing service close to the battlefield (McEnroe, 2012).

The final feature of this schema of resilience is possessing a spirit of optimism and hope that things will change (Hill, 1960). This type of person continues to aspire to reach goals despite the obstacles in the way. Australian nurse Elizabeth Kenny is an example of this kind of resilience in action. Before the First World War, Kenny was working as an unqualified nurse in a cottage hospital near the small town of Guyra in New South Wales. It was there that she encountered numerous cases of infantile paralysis. After volunteering to work as a nurse in the war she received rigorous training working on troopships, earning promotion to Sister and eventually returning to regional nursing, where a polio epidemic was then raging.

The conventional treatment, which involved immobilizing bodies in plaster casts, was ineffective, and so Kenny found ways to work with doctors to enable her treatment of exercise and hot compresses to be used instead. Despite resistance from many in the medical community, Kenny persisted in her belief about this course of treatment and, due to her efforts, was instrumental in establishing numerous clinics that successfully utilized her methods. In 2009, her treatment was duly, but tardily, recognized as one of the 150 Queensland icons of innovation and invention achieved throughout the century and a half of the State's history (Rogers, 2013)

While resiliency is a positive personal attribute, and these inspiring historical examples of extraordinary nursing heroism are important to recognize, such examples have a tendency to both individualize and internalize the issue. Strength is seen as existing in one special nurse, and thus the nurse is idealized and rarified. The strengths this nurse possesses are assumed to be unique to his or her genetic, family, or personal makeup. These stories, and the hero worship of such figures (no matter how deserved), also obscures the reality that social competence may have contributed to these individuals' abilities to cope, and that coping may not, in itself, be an appropriate long-term solution to deal with the adversities of life and work. Indeed, focusing on, and expecting, individuals to make such extraordinary reactions in such situations does nothing to eradicate the problems that lie at the source of these issues, and that may allow problems to percolate and worsen. This can, moreover, ultimately accumulate as trauma for not only the nurses involved, but also future nurses who have to work in, and through, the situations and conditions that have been caused and enshrined by such idolization.

This means that there are a number of flaws in utilizing such a psychological, and now normative (i.e., one which has become so widely understood as to be seen as best practice), model of resilience (Pratt, 2015). This is summed up by Traynor's (2017, p. 28) somewhat sardonic observation, "resilience thinking is often about bouncing back to where you were before something bad happens, but what if where you were sucks?" A view of resilience that focuses on a nurse developing individual traits and abilities to cope with the working situation obscures the structural factors that exist to impede not only that nurse's but all of contemporary nursing's effectiveness and potential, as well as its ability to generate and sustain a positive identity. In this, nurses—and everyone else—who subscribe to the idea that it is an individual's responsibility to take sole charge of staying strong and upbeat, reinforce a belief that society is made up of individuals each working to maximize their individual potential. They also (often unthinkingly) negate the idea that the situation that is requiring that strength and positivity can be changed or improved.

*Resiliency is the psychological capacity to withstand or bounce back from adversity.*

*Resilience is the psychosocial capacity to use adversity to spur renewal and innovative thinking.*

Neocleous (2013) agrees, arguing that resilience has been co-opted into the economic and social imperatives of contemporary neoliberalism. In this understanding of the way the world works, individuals look inward to the self and its resources, rather than confronting social injustice and hardships. Thus, resilience interventions tend to focus on encouraging individuals to think positively to cope and to employ self-help strategies (Jackson, Fau-Firtko, & Edenborough, 2007). This means that limited, or no, structural changes or solutions will be forthcoming, and the situation may well worsen. This results in an ever downward spiral whereby individuals work harder and harder to cope with adverse situations that only allow the situation to continue to deteriorate, thus necessitating more work to cope.

Many nurses appear to be incapable to resist this cycle. Indeed, at times, they function as what Zizek (2005) terms "righteous victims." Nurses are righteous victims when they find pleasure in repeating accounts of their powerlessness because it allows them to take the moral high ground in adverse situations. Evidence of nurses acting in this way can be seen when they accept extra patient or student loads or extra tasks or hours and soldier on, rather than protest (Fealy & McNamara, 2015). Such resistance is also anathema to that entrenched virtue script begun with Florence Nightingale of doing one's duty and being selfless and focused on the other. While this sounds admirable, it is a risky practice, for what is to stop those extra loads continuing to increase, and increase yet again, to breaking point?

In addition, the risks of being overworked, and acquiescing in this, are becoming starkly apparent, and can no longer be ignored, even by the most neo-liberal of employers. Reports of healthcare failings have, for example, been directly linked to over work (Francis, 2013), with numerous studies reporting the consequences. Expressed most simply: The higher the workload, the lower the quality of patient care (Aiken et al., 2013). Overwork is also the most intensely experienced stressor for nurses and other healthcare professionals (Poulsen et al., 2014) and is directly related to high and increasing rates of workplace bullying, dissatisfaction, burnout, and turnover rates (Khamisa, Peltzer, & Oldenburg, 2013; Leon Perez, Medina, Arenas, & Munduate, 2015; McCann et al., 2013; Sharp, McAllister, & Broadbent, 2016). Ironically, this overwork is frequently caused not even by legitimate patient care, but by what is often called "busywork" (that which keeps a worker busy but has little or no real or actual value, and which Covey (2004, p. 151) would characterize as unimportant nonurgent activities) such as restocking of a treatment cupboard, or support service satisfaction surveys. When so consumed with what can be identified as such busy-work, some nurses have failed to see patient needs. This "inattentive blindness," as Zimbardo (2007) puts it, is what happened with the hundreds of nurses implicated in the Staffordshire hospital scandal. Patients repeatedly complained of being neglected, yet nurses did not respond compassionately or effectively (Francis, 2013). It appears they did not because they were overwhelmed with completing other tasks (including paperwork) that was demanded of them.

Clearly, many nurses, managers, and health planners fail to recognize that the social and cultural context in which nursing work occurs has an impact—and a significant impact—on patients' progress, the course of their suffering, and their recovery (Paley, 2014). This reveals that nurses are not well skilled in what can be described as structural competence (Metzl & Hansen, 2014). Structural competence is the ability to recognize the part that social structures, such as various inequities (around class, gender, and age, for instance) and living and working conditions, play in influencing health and well-being. Ironically, nurses' overdeveloped desire to be demure and untroublesome only serves to confirm the hegemonic virtue script in which they have been so well trained (as described earlier in this chapter), but this actually hampers their ability to be the most capable and effective carers they could be.

*Resilience is not just reactive, but proactive. Knowing that adversity, tension, or dilemmas could be ahead provides opportunity for marshalling resources, and cognitive rehearsal.*

So, rather than think of resilience, which involves the ability to roll with the punches—and retrospectively dealing with hardships and adversity—we, instead, suggest that a better, and more productive and sustainable, form of resilience involves the ability to examine, and develop, ways to avoid getting hit in the first place. This form of active, forward-facing resilience requires a series of actions. These are understanding the contributors to stress in the environment, working collectively to challenge and change what is unacceptable and—rather than suppress negative feelings and simply trying to cope—to see these as physical signals that require attention and action. In contrast to the individualistic and even dangerous definition of resilience stated earlier, a more fitting definition is provided by the Stockholm Resilience Centre. In these terms, resilience is "the capacity of a system to use shocks and disturbances . . . to spur renewal and innovative thinking" (Stockholm Resilience Centre, 2012, p. 3).

## RESILIENCE CAN BE LEARNED

### Dispute Pessimistic Thinking

Various disciplines have now produced convincing evidence that individuals can learn resilience and acquire resilient qualities. This means that strength does not solely depend on the natural talents of the individuals involved. The positive psychology movement has been a leader in this research. Seligman's (2006) work on learned optimism, for example, argues that a person's explanatory style (how individuals explain to themselves why they experience events) shapes the meaning and the effect of adverse experiences. Moreover, one can learn to be optimistic by using focused cognitive behavioral techniques that dispute pessimistic thinking and allow the individual to become more adaptive and resilient. Performing exercises to identify and dispute such negative thinking can assist here (see the ABCDE exercise in Box 4.1).

## BOX 4.1 Disputing Pessimistic Thinking: ABCDE Exercise

1. Write down the nature of the ADVERSITY
2. Identify any negative BELIEFS triggered by the problem
3. Record the CONSEQUENCE of the problem, how you are feeling and acting as a result
4. DISPUTE the negative belief, challenging it, thinking of other possible reasons for the problem
5. Consider the more optimistic EXPLANATIONS for your problem

### Learn How to Reflect

Reflection is a familiar concept in everyday life. It is often taken to mean "to look back." It is also a common activity requested of students by educators in nursing. Certainly reflection can help one to look again at a situation and to find new ways of dealing with it. Reflection is vital for the resilient person.

However, in learning, reflection has potential to mean something deeper that simply looking back, and when it is practiced to its fullest extent, it has been shown to help a person self-correct, cease making the same cognitive/emotional or practical errors that lead to negative outcomes, and to open up to a new worldview (Mezirow, 2000). A clear definition of reflection is that it is the art of pondering on one's virtues and flaws.

*Reflection is the art of pondering on one's virtues and flaws.*

Consider these examples. Jamie realized she kept getting her dosage calculations wrong, so she reflected on where the stumbling block was, sought help to have that step re-explained, and now gets the drug calculations right every time.

Susan was thinking about a significant event that happened in emergency, where a distressed young mother (like Susan) came in with her child who was unconscious, having slipped into the backyard pool. Susan became upset, too, and could barely hold it together to complete her tasks. She realized she empathized with this mother too much and needed to learn a way to distance herself sufficiently to be objective and emotionally contained in such situations.

Paul was an experienced politician who held narrow views about a minority group that others told him were racist. He was taken on a guided excursion for a television show, where finally he got to meet the families of this minority, to talk with them, and to see things from their point of view. He experienced an epiphany and totally changed his perspective. Now he is an advocate for this community.

Notice that different kinds of reflection and change are going on in these scenarios. How have each of these people changed? Jamie has learned to use a different kind of cognitive process—to seek support to problem solve. Susan has learned about her emotions and searched for another way to cope. The first two people looked back on their actions. They reflected on action. Jamie reflected on thought. Susan reflected on feelings.

Unlike Jamie and Susan, Paul reflected in practice. He also reflected on the feelings of others. Something happened that was quite transformative and he realized that past views were ill-fitting and inaccurate. In listening, talking, asking questions, he put his own ideas aside and gradually his accepted truths were replaced. He engaged in some unlearning.

Reflection is the process of analyzing, questioning, and reframing an experience in order to make an assessment of it for the purposes of learning (reflective learning) and/or to improve practice (reflective practice).

There are many ways to reflect and, to ensure you are in the mood to reflect, it is important to be away from the work context, feeling relaxed and not emotionally activated or defensive, so that your mind is ready to ponder and to think creatively. Aronson (2011) suggests these six strategies:

1. Link past, present, and future experiences; for example, *The stress began here, the same thing cropped up just now, and it will again if I don't do something differently*
2. Integrate cognitive and emotional reactions; for example, *What was the problem, how did I react?*

3. Consider the experience from multiple perspectives; for example, *What would Gandhi or Mother Teresa or an "admired other" have made of this event?*
4. Try reframing; for example, *This crisis was an opportunity.*
5. State the lesson learned; for example, *The moral of that story was "Trust your instincts."*
6. Plan for future learning or practice; for example, *In future, I will try to make friends early because they will be sources of support*

## Keep a Journal

Nurses encounter serious events every day in their practice, sometimes one after the other! There is often very little time to reflect on each one as they occur. This is why keeping a daily journal or blog, where you note down what happened, can help. You can come back to it later and reflect on it so that you learn from any errors you made at the time, and also praise yourself for the virtues you showed during a time of stress. Self-critique and self-validation are two important ways to engage in self-care.

## Uncover Habits of Mind

Brookfield (1990) explains that self-critique requires us to look below the surface of our own actions, to bring to the surface unconscious habits or biases that we may have buried, or never looked at because they came to us from school or family or media, in a kind of script already written. When we self-critique, we may uncover habits of mind that could be reframed (Costa & Kallick, 2000; Table 4.1).

## Analyze Significant Events

If we get into the habit of self-critique after work, when the emotional intensity of the event has lessened, we can be more analytical of ourselves and ready to develop. On the other hand, if something serious happens at work, and we decide to have a drink to forget it, there is a risk that the issue will not be processed and it may continue to replay in your mind. This can lead to trauma (van der Kolk, 2003). By reflecting using the significant incident technique, one can look at the situation with some distance and objectivity. Figure 4.1 shows a process for analyzing significant events.

Table 4.1  Habits of Mind

| Habits of Mind | |
| --- | --- |
| **Unconsciously Used and Often Ineffective** | **Consciously Used and Effective** |
| Negative self-talk<br>• *I'm not capable*<br>• *I don't have what it takes*<br>• *I was wrong before, I'll be wrong again*<br>Emotions take the lead<br>• Fear, panic, avoidance<br>• Defensive<br>• Frustrated, tearful, angry<br>Defeatist self-talk<br>• *It won't work*<br>• *Life's not fair*<br>Blaming<br>• Other people are the problem<br>• Self-abuse<br>Magical thinking<br>• I can guess what they're thinking<br>• It's just like last time<br>• If it's meant to happen, it will | Positive self-talk<br>• *I love a challenge*<br>• *Onward and upward*<br>• *I can do this*<br>Thinking takes the lead<br>• Persisting<br>• Thinking and communicating with clarity and precision<br>• Managing impulsivity<br>• Gathering data through all senses<br>Listening with understanding and empathy<br>Creating, imagining, innovating<br>Taking responsible risks<br>Finding humor<br>Questioning<br>Thinking interdependently<br>Applying past knowledge to new situations<br>Remaining open to new learning |

Perhaps one might find the need for more problem-solving strategies, or maybe a wider range of self-soothing mechanisms. We also might need to think about the feelings of others more or take the time to look at preceding events that added to the situation that could be dealt with differently next time.

The idea is to think about an event that happened that was challenging, adverse, or momentous. Describe what happened. You could then move on to think or talk about what happened next. For example: What did you do? What reactions did you and others have to the event? What feelings were evoked? Or, you could move back from the happening to think about what happened before the event that perhaps precipitated it. Were there a series of small events that occurred? Did it come out of the blue? What were the contributing factors?

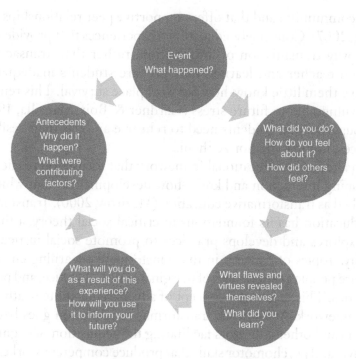

**Figure 4.1** Significant incident analysis.

*Source:* Adapted from Brookfield, S. D. (1990). Using critical incidents to explore learners' assumptions. In J. Mezirow (Ed.), *Fostering critical reflection in adulthood* (pp. 177–193). San Francisco, CA: Jossey-Bass.

Once you have examined the impact on self and others, what virtues and flaws in your response style became apparent? Did you use effective and conscious habits of mind, or did you resort to pre-existing and unconscious reactionary styles? Did you have a knowledge gap that needs to be filled? Would you benefit from social support structures in future?

Now that you have analyzed your strengths and weaknesses, it's time to learn from the event. What will you do differently as a result of this experience? What will happen next time?

## Teaching Contexts That Are Learner Centered

Within the educational context, evidence suggests that resilience can be improved through the development of relevant and practical protective factors. These include an educational setting that is caring and learner-centered; that has positive, high expectations; provides a positive learning environment; is placed within a strong, supportive, social community; and that offers supportive peer relationships (Gu & Day, 2007). Conversely, educational experiences that provide only a one-way transmission of information, rather than transactions between teacher and learner, may prepare students inadequately and give them little know-how for workplace survival. This renders them vulnerable to future stress (Gardner & Boix-Mansilla, 1999). This suggests that students need to rehearse and use their resilient practices, not just memorize them.

An alternative educational framework that focuses on resilience-developing interaction and know-how development is that which is described as transformative education (Mezirow, 2000). Transformative education has its foundations in critical social theory, a theory that explores and develops practices to promote social justice and equality. Topics of concern in the transformative learning environment are people's experiences of marginalization, injustice, and power inequities. This means the concept of adversity fits quite neatly into this framework. At its heart, transformative education goes beyond teachers and other educators facilitating the acquisition of cognitive, affective, and psychomotor skills that produce competent workers, to provide training that produces critical, empowered (and empowering) knowledge workers. Instead, it seeks to use critical and constructive thinking methods to inspire learners to look deeply into practices, develop creative ways of thinking, improve their problem-solving, and strive to further social good through their personal actions. Learning resilience fits well within the transformative educational framework.

In such transformative learning, learning from the insights of individual health professionals and relating these insights to well-being is also important. In addition, the clinician's orientation to the nature of the work and how meaningful it is to their own life is also significant. If the work is "just a job" (as it is for some clinicians), then this viewpoint may be correlated with lower levels of resilience. Researching how clinicians process and understand experiences that are significant and even traumatic, such as the first time they face an untimely death of a patient, could also yield valuable information. Understanding the coping styles and capabilities that clinicians bring to their work, gained either through genetic or environmental factors, may well help others understand what helps those clinicians endure challenges and even grow from them. We can put this style of learning to work by examining a story from nursing's history that has been portrayed in a major film.

## LEARNING FROM HISTORICAL EXAMPLES

*Paradise Road* (Beresford, 1997) is one of the few films where nurses are represented as a group rather than (a series of) individuals. This is, moreover, a group that is tested in a crisis and that responds collectively in innovative and inspiring ways. Set during the Second World War, at the time of the fall of Singapore, this is the fact-based story of a group of women who were interned in a prisoner of war camp in the jungles of Sumatra. Some were the survivors of the bombed British ship the *Vyner Brooke*. These survivors included Australian army nurses, Dutch women who had been living in the East Indies, English women from Singapore, missionaries, Catholic nuns, and others from diverse nations, races, and positions in society. They were captured, imprisoned, and endured deprivation and harsh treatment before being freed 3 years later when the Japanese surrendered. The director, Bruce Beresford, stated that the film was based on the diaries of Sister Betty Jeffrey, published in *White Coolies* (Jeffrey, 1958), and the testimonies of many Japanese prisoner of war survivors, including nursing sister Vivian Bullwinkel.

In contrast to other stories of resilience, the nurses in this film do not turn inward and focus on themselves. Instead, they turn to each other for support and, in doing so, find that their united strength is what helps each person deal with the adversity. As such, this becomes a film about how small, repeated, externally focused resistance practices not only enable individuals to cope with trauma, but how it also assists them to reclaim some sense of power and, then, to refuse seeing themselves as victims.

Although the women are culturally divided—there are language, religious, political, and social barriers—they make a decision early in their imprisonment to look out for one another. In one powerful scene, Susan Macarthy, played by Cate Blanchett, after defying an order for silence, is forced to kneel in the open air under the blaze of the tropical sun for many hours. She is humiliated, demoralized, and her already weakened state is pushed to its limits. But upon her release, she is immediately tended to by her comrades. She is fed, cleaned, and her wounds tended to. Others take up her duties until she is well again. When starving and forced to eat rancid rice, one of the women catches a snake in the paddy field and the others help to cook it and distribute the result. They are all individually weak and vulnerable, but each gains strength by sharing the workload. When one in the group is rewarded with a gift of soap, she shares it with the others and, in this way, when one woman benefits, they all do. The film is also unusual in not depicting any one clear leader of the group, although numerous characters demonstrate leadership skills that together work to meet everyone's physical and emotional needs. For example, one Dutch woman, who is clearly well educated and higher class than many of the others, uses her cunning to barter with the guards and secure medicines, alcohol, and food. Although not trusted by all of the women, she contributes by liaising with the nurses to distribute her meager goods.

At the center of the plot is a kind of a choir, whereby the women use their voices to produce a vocal orchestra, as they have no other instruments. This serves many resilience functions for the women. It is a mechanism that allows them to transcend their suffering, for they are each focused on learning and performing their parts and contributing meaningfully to the choir so that each song succeeds. A simple distraction from the adverse conditions, the choir also gives the women power. By singing, they are refusing to be suppressed, or to succumb to the gross dehumanization of the camp. The women become singers, rather than faceless, walking corpses. They are thus engaged in an exercise of soft power—power that serves needs and desires yet does not oppress. It also models to others, including their Japanese jailers, a higher form of being human than the destructive approach exemplified by their captors.

*The strength-giving power of resilience can involve distraction, humor, transcendence, and soft power.*

There is an important scene of conflict in the film, when the group threatens to divide. The young attractive women are invited to live in the Japanese officers' club where they will enjoy good food, clean rooms, hot water, and leisure, in return for providing the men with sexual favors. Many of the women are horrified and repulsed, but some find the offer too tempting to refuse. Instead of causing irreparable fragmentation in the group, those who stay joke that they will "starve and sing," and do not judge their sisters who have chosen this (also) very difficult path of survival. While all the women do face the reality that they may be doomed, they do not give up on life. This fortitude is encapsulated in an important scene toward the end of the film in which the choir director, frail and dying, shares a final word of wisdom with her comrades, which gives them courage, moral power, and purpose. She says, "I can't hate them. The worse they behave, the sorrier I feel for them." This sense is also evident in the film's title of *Paradise Road*, which refers to the journey toward death, which is inevitable for each of those living. Along the way, this journey may be in turn sublimely beautiful or terrifyingly horrendous. In this way, this film echoes the words made famous by Viktor Frankl, the Holocaust survivor, psychiatrist, and philosopher, who stated that "Everything can be taken from a man but one thing: the last of the human freedoms—to choose one's attitude in any given set of circumstances, to choose one's own way" (Frankl, 1985, p. 86).

## LEARNING TO APPLY THE RESILIENCE STANDPOINT

Instead of the women in this story becoming self-focused, or the group disintegrating into cliques, they bond as a group, and it is the strength of shared purpose, empathy, and support that enables the group to endure, retain hope, adapt, and continue to act outwardly. This is, thus, an extreme example of how reliance can be sourced via community involvement and actions. Within this group, no single individual leads all the time, attempts to speak for everyone, or possesses all the necessary qualities to steer the group politically, physically, or emotionally. Instead, each person is shown to have unique strengths that are co-opted and put to use to foster the resilience, and resulting well-being, of the group. This distributes risk and also allows each individual to find a niche and be of use for the good of the group. While some members are (or become) more vulnerable than others, their collective strength helps them maintain hope, direction, and—in turn—provides a model of acting that can be internalized and personally owned. Individuals who may otherwise have given up find the courage to endure. In this way, the group becomes more than the sum of its individual parts, and there is a clear reason to maintain one's membership. This is an example of how resilience involves harnessing unique capabilities.

*Resilience in nursing involves cultivating strong teams, collegial support, and standing firm together.*

The nurses and the other women in this story creatively respond to, and cope with, their situation. When there is no food, they find it. When there is no medicine, they trade. When others attempt to dehumanize them, they reclaim their humanity. In the face of violence, they enact nonviolent resistance. While they are not able to manage the adversity at its source (i.e., by vanquishing their jailers), they do not simply "roll with the punches." Whenever they can, they exert their power by refusing the status of victim, and by acting in ways that show they are actually stronger than their enemy. This also illustrates how resilience involves accessing cultural resources that emphasize humanity.

The women make their everyday work bearable by sharing jokes, telling stories, and offering small words of encouragement to each other. Their choir demonstrates their skill, focus, shared labor, and determination to access the cultural resources that can give them back identity, beauty, and spiritual connection. What these nurses and other women did was to routinize the traumatic—something that the nursing literature says is a common practice for many nurses because their everyday work involves so much suffering and trauma. This routinizing of the traumatic lessens the emotional cadence and assists in making unbearable work more bearable (Chambliss, 1996). These are all examples of how resilience involves outward social actions.

*More than simply internal, psychological traits, resilience in nursing involves outward social actions aimed at keeping the patient, and the profession, strong and capable.*

Connected to the determination to maintain their humanity, and refusal to be internally divided, is the part in the story where, while some of the women made the decision to become "comfort women" to the Japanese soldiers, the remaining prisoners suspended judgment about this choice. This is an example of how resilience sometimes rests in acceptance. Learning when to use resilience tactics, when to resist and when to just pause, is part of the dynamic process of resilience.

## IMPLICATIONS OF A RESILENCE STANDPOINT FOR THE NURSING ROLE

Possessing an explicit resilience standpoint, as did the women in *Paradise Road*, is helpful in guiding the way that nurses encourage and support patients. First, nurses should assess the strengths that exist in the person they are nursing, as well as the patient's family and environment. They should then then aim to utilize these strengths so that they can operate as support structures during the illness and recovery process. Educating patients about the benefits of developing a wide repertoire of coping mechanisms may be very useful in raising awareness of resilience. Explaining healthy coping mechanisms and developing a relevant list with clients can be helpful. Such strategies might include exercise, yoga, meditation, conversation, reading, listening to music, looking at photographs, or using applications of heat or cold. Encouraging patients by identifying realistic short-term goals and then commenting positively on progress made and what is being achieved can cultivate hope and optimism for the future.

There are also practices that nurses can engage in to contribute to a happier and healthier work culture. Health environments can be notoriously bureaucratic and hierarchical, and both new and continuing nurses are likely to experience ideological tensions, power inequities, and ethical dilemmas. Vulnerable newcomers may especially experience self-doubt and tentativeness, and a lack of connectedness in their workplace. More experienced nurses can facilitate a sense of belonging in new staff members by welcoming them, appreciating that any timidness, aloofness, and tendency to require solitude on a new nurse's part may indicate a lack of confidence and signal the need for displays of kindness and friendliness. Experienced nurses can also encourage newcomers to ask questions in ways that are not abrupt or confronting but are instead expressed out of curiosity and a desire to learn. This builds trust and rapport among staff and also encourages newcomers to be change agents and critical thinkers (McAllister, Tower, & Walker, 2007).

New nurses also benefit from exposure to positive role models who can share strategies on how to thrive in health workplaces. Such imitative learning is a powerful learning strategy (Bandura, 1975). More experienced nurses who thus act as "teachers" will also benefit, because their sense of generativity will grow. Generativity, or altruism, is a resilience attribute and involves giving back to the new generation and continuing to make a positive contribution to the culture, no matter what advanced stage of career has been reached. Enabling and valuing such generativity in the workplace also makes better use of the nursing profession's elders and helps them to feel fulfilled, which is (in itself) an asset for the profession. There are many ways to enable generativity. For example, resilient clinicians can be encouraged to share lessons learned from their own experience for the benefit of the future workforce through such dialogical activities as shared storytelling at seminars and conferences and via publications and creative expression such as poetry, art, autobiographical writing, and film making.

Nurses can, themselves, powerfully reorient their practice to be strengths-based, simply by changing the way they speak to, and about, clients. For instance, a health assessment could include a question like, "What are your hobbies, talents, and strengths?"

Then, to be instructive, the nurse could suggest, "Can you please select two or three of these so that together we can work out how they might be incorporated into your health planning and speed your recovery?" Also, instead of focusing on the identifying risks that the client may be exposed to, this can be reframed to consider safety. Instead of, "What is the risk of self-harm or suicide for this client?," nurses could ask, "How can our service promote this client's psychological safety?"

Leaders and managers can also develop a less bureaucratic decision-making style so that their workforce feels involved and therefore more loyal to the workplace. Some strategies to do this include:

1. Actively supporting time away from hands-on nursing so that thinking time is possible. This time can be used for positive role modeling and to support reflection on practice. Such sessions could also focus on helping nurses to find meaning in challenging situations (How did their role make a difference?), increasing manageability (How can these situations be managed

better next time?), and a more thorough comprehension of experiences (Why did this happen in the way it did?).

2. Managers can invite experienced nurses to act as mentors to new staff and develop a relationship where the new staff feel comfortable in interrupting poor practices.

3. Finally, this resilience-based thinking should be applied by nurses and others to field research so that the effectiveness of nurse-led interventions can be established, and so that more evidence-based interventions can be developed.

## IMPLICATIONS FOR NURSING EDUCATION

An important goal for educators is to build strengths that equip students with interpersonal and psychosocial strategies to assist them in making a successful transition to the health workplace, prepare them for the pressures and challenges of the work environment, and encourage their social activism to build more inclusive, supportive workplaces. Resilience is relevant to everyone's well-being, and since nurses and nursing students may be particularly vulnerable because of the stress they experience, it ought to be a concept that is taught in engaging and memorable ways. Developing a confident, proud identity can build self-belief and a calm demeanor under stress (King, Newman, & Luthans, 2016). Therefore, discussions of positive role models in nursing, and inclusion of nursing history so that students can see how far nursing has developed and what obstacles have already been overcome, can develop a sense of social connectedness and belonging. Asking students what they believe in, what their aims are, and what they intend to contribute to the world, are all strategies to develop a sense of professional commitment and optimism.

It is also vital that students are responsibly prepared for the reality of the stressors and potential for adversity that are common within complex health systems. One way to do this is to include resilience in the curriculum and to engage students in *reflection for practice*. This involves prompting students to consider and brainstorm such questions as the following:

1. What strengths and supports can I use to help me during stressful times at work?

2. What coping skills have I used effectively in the past to cope with stressful situations? How can I extend my repertoire?
3. What do I need to know about what it takes to succeed in practice?
4. What am I likely to encounter in hospitals and health centers that I need to be prepared for?
5. How can I develop critical and creative thinking skills, and a sense of humor, to help me transcend difficulties?
6. What can I do when I am on clinical placement that may help to contribute to a happy, collaborative atmosphere among the team?

Another strategy to build a sense of professional belonging—and thus resilience—is to provide a forum where a range of students, nurses, and sympathetic community members can come together to exchange ideas and celebrate the positive achievements of nursing. These could be held around such important calendar dates as International Nurses' Day, for instance, and could include guest speakers to discuss landmark moments in nursing's history or photography competitions that invite students to make positive images of nursing that can be shared with the local media (McAllister et al., 2011).

## CONCLUSION

Rather than think of resilience as the ability to bounce back to where you once were when faced with adversity, resilience can be thought of as doing what is needed to survive, and even develop and thrive, in difficult situations. Adverse experiences are never ideal, but they can lead to personal growth and change. The resilience standpoint that we propose in this chapter is one that challenges the taken-for-granted idea that resilience is an individual state involving cognitive flexibility, optimism, and stress hardiness. Instead, we suggest that resilience can be learned and developed by disputing pessimistic thoughts, learning how to reflect, challenge habits of mind, and analyze significant events so they are processed and resolved. It is also important to draw on the power of the group. An active ongoing membership of, and positive contribution to, that group can allow individuals to internalize and develop hidden strengths and, ultimately, to flourish, despite difficult and adverse working conditions.

## LEARNING ACTIVITIES

1. Bruce Beresford's Film *Paradise Road* is a fictionalized rendering of a true story in nursing's history. Respond to this statement by drawing on examples within the film to explain your argument:

Encountering conflict is an inevitable facet of human existence. The film highlights the potential of conflict to catalyze the revaluation of an individual's moral compass, the way in which one lives, and the values that are important to their existence to be realized.

2. Construct a palm card to summarize the resilience standpoint that you could give to patients or use yourself.

## REFERENCES

Aiken, L. H., Sloane, D. M., Bruyneel, L., Van den Heede, K., Sermeus, W., & Rn4cast Consortium. (2013). Nurses' reports of working conditions and hospital quality of care in 12 countries in Europe. *International Journal of Nursing Studies, 50*(2), 143–153. doi:10.1016/j.ijnurstu.2012.11.009

Aronson, L. (2011). Twelve tips for teaching reflection at all levels of medical education. *Medical Teacher, 33*(3), 200–205. doi:10.3109/0142159X.2010.507714

Bandura, A. (1975). Analysis of modeling processes. *School Psychology Digest, 4*(1), 4–10.

Beresford, B. (Dir). (1997). *Paradise Road.* Sydney, Australia: Samson Productions.

Brookfield, S. D. (1990). Using critical incidents to explore learners' assumptions. In J. Mezirow (Ed.), *Fostering critical reflection in adulthood* (pp. 177–193). San Francisco, CA: Jossey-Bass.

Chambliss, D. F. (1996). *Beyond caring: Hospitals, nurses, and the social organization of ethics.* Chicago, IL: University of Chicago Press.

Costa, A., & Kallick, B. (2000). *Discovering and exploring habits of mind. A developmental series, Book 1.* Alexandria, VA: Association for Supervision and Curriculum Development.

Covey, S. (2004). *The 7 habits of highly effective people: Powerful lessons in personal change.* New York, NY: Free Press.

Diertele, W. (Dir). (1936). *The white angel.* Burbank, CA: Warner Bros.

Fealy, G., & McNamara, M. (2015). Transitions and tensions: The discipline of nursing in an interdisciplinary context. *Journal of Nursing Management, 23*(1), 1–3. doi:10.1111/jonm.12282

Forrester, D. (2016). *Nursing's greatest leaders: A history of activism.* New York, NY: Springer Publishing Company.

Francis, R. (2013). *Report of the Mid Staffordshire NHS Foundation Trust public inquiry: Executive summary (Vol. 947).* London, UK: The Stationery Office.

Frankl, V. E. (1985). *Man's search for meaning*. London, UK: Simon and Schuster.

Gardner, H., & Boix-Mansilla, V. (1999). Teaching for understanding in the disciplines–and beyond. *Learners and Pedagogy*, 78–88.

Gordon, S., & Nelson, S. (2006). Moving beyond the virtue script in nursing: Creating a knowledge-based identity for nurses. In S. Nelson & S. Gordon (Eds.), *The complexities of care: Nursing reconsidered* (pp.13–29). New York, NY: Cornell University Press.

Gu, Q., & Day, C. (2007). Teachers resilience: A necessary condition for effectiveness. *Teaching and Teacher Education, 23*(8), 1302–1316. doi:10.1016/j.tate.2006.06.006

Harding, S. G. (Ed.). (2004). *The feminist standpoint theory reader: Intellectual and political controversies*. Abingdon, UK: Psychology Press.

Hill, N. (1960). *Think and grow rich* (Rev. ed.). Greenwich, CT: Fawcett Crest.

Jackson, D., Fau-Firtko, A., & Edenborough, M. (2007). Personal resilience as a strategy for surviving and thriving in the face of workplace adversity: A literature review. *Journal of Advanced Nursing, 60*(1), 1–9. doi:10.1111/j.1365-2648.2007.04412.x

Jeffrey, B. (1958). *White coolies*. Sydney, Australia: Panther.

Kelly, J., Fealy, G., & Watson, R. (2012). The image of you: Constructing nursing identities in YouTube. *Journal of Advanced Nursing, 68*(8), 1804–1813. doi:10.1111/j.1365-2648.2011.05872.x

Khamisa, N., Peltzer, K., & Oldenburg, B. (2013). Burnout in relation to specific contributing factors and health outcomes among nurses: A systematic review. *International Journal of Environmental Research and Public Health, 10*(6), 2214–2240. doi:10.3390/ijerph10062214

King, D. D., Newman, A., & Luthans, F. (2016). Not if, but when we need resilience in the workplace. *Journal of Organizational Behavior, 37*(5), 782–786. doi:10.1002/job.2063

Kobasa, S. C. (1979). Stressful life events, personality, and health—Inquiry into hardiness. *Journal of Personality and Social Psychology, 37*(1), 1–11. doi:10.1037/0022-3514.37.1.1

Leon Perez, J., Medina, F., Arenas, A., & Munduate, L. (2015). The relationship between interpersonal conflict and workplace bullying. *Journal of Managerial Psychology, 30*(3), 250–263. doi:10.1108/JMP-01-2013-0034

Levett-Jones, T., & Lathlean, J. (2009). "Don't rock the boat": Nursing students' experiences of conformity and compliance. *Nurse Education Today, 29*(3), 342–349. doi:10.1016/j.nedt.2008.10.009

McAllister, M., Tower, M., & Walker, R. (2007). Gentle interruptions: Transformative approaches to clinical teaching. *Journal of Nursing Education, 46*(7), 304–313.

McAllister, M., Williams, L., Hope, J., Hallett, C., Framp, A., Doyle, B., & McLeod, M. (2011). In my day II: Reflecting on the transformative potential of incorporating celebrations into the nursing curriculum. *Nurse Education in Practice, 11*(4), 245–249. doi:10.1016/j.nepr.2010.11.014

McCann, C., Beddoe, E., McCormick, K., Huggard, P., Kedge, S., Adamson, C., & Huggard, J. (2013). Resilience in the health professions. A review of the current literature. *International Journal of Wellbeing, 3*(1), 60–81. doi:10.5502/ijw.v3i1.4

McEnroe, N. (2012, September 3). Beyond the rivalry: Florence Nightingale and Mary Seacole. *History Today*. Retrieved from https://www.historytoday.com/beyond-rivalry-florence-nightingale-and-mary-seacole

Metzl, J. M., & Hansen, H. (2014). Structural competency: Theorizing a new medical engagement with stigma and inequality. *Social Science & Medicine, 103*, 126–133. doi:10.1016/j.socscimed.2013.06.032

Meyer, B. C., & Bishop, D. S. (2007). Florence Nightingale: Nineteenth century apostle of quality. *Journal of Management History, 13*(3), 240–254. doi:10.1108/17511340710754699

Mezirow, J. (2000). *Learning as transformation: Critical perspectives on a theory in progress. The Jossey-Bass Higher and Adult Education Series.* San Francisco, CA: Jossey-Bass.

Neocleous, M. (2013). Resisting resilience. *Radical Philosophy, 178*, 2–7.

Paley, J. (2014). Cognition and the compassion deficit: The social psychology of helping behaviour in nursing. *Nursing Philosophy, 15*(4), 274–287. doi:10.1111/nup.12047

Poulsen, A. A., Meredith, P., Khan, A., Henderson, J., Castrisos, V., & Khan, S. R. (2014). Burnout and work engagement in occupational therapists. *British Journal of Occupational Therapy, 77*(3), 156–164. doi:10.4276/030802214X13941036266621

Pratt, A. C. (2015). Resilience, locality and the cultural economy. *City, Culture and Society, 6*(3), 61–67. doi:10.1016/j.ccs.2014.11.001

Rogers, N. (2013). *Polio wars: Sister Kenny and the golden age of American medicine.* Oxford, UK: Oxford University Press.

Rotter, J. (1966). Generalized expectancies for internal versus external control of reinforcement. *Psychological Monographs: General & Applied. 80*(1), 1–28. doi:10.1037/h0092976

Seligman, M. E. (2006). *Learned optimism: How to change your mind and your life.* New York, NY: Vintage.

Sharp, S., McAllister, M., & Broadbent, M. (2016). The vital blend of clinical competence and compassion: How patients experience person-centred care. *Contemporary Nurse, 51*(2), 1–13. doi:10.1080/10376178.2015.1020981

Stanley, D. (2008). Celluloid angels: A research study of nurses in feature films 1900-2007. *Journal of Advanced Nursing, 64*(1), 84–95. doi:10.1111/j.1365-2648.2008.04793.x

Stockholm Resilience Centre. (2012). Retrieved from http://www.stockholmresilience.org

Traynor, M. (2017). *Critical resilience for nurses: An evidence-based guide to survival and change in the modern NHS.* London, UK: Routledge.

Tugade, M. M., & Fredrickson, B. L. (2004). Resilient individuals use positive emotions to bounce back from negative emotional experiences. *Journal of Personality and Social Psychology, 86*(2), 320–333. doi:10.1037/0022-3514.86.2.320

Tugade, M. M., Fredrickson, B. L., & Feldman Barrett, L. (2004). Psychological resilience and positive emotional granularity: Examining the benefits of positive emotions on coping and health. *Journal of Personality, 72*(6), 1161–1190. doi:10.1111/j.1467-6494.2004.00294.x

Van der Kolk, B. A. (2003). *Psychological trauma*. Philadelphia, PA: American Psychiatric Association.

Zimbardo, P. (2007). *The Lucifer effect: How good people turn evil*. London, UK: Rider.

Zizek, S. (2005). *Beyond discourse analysis. Interrogating the real* (pp. 271–284). London, UK: Continuum.

# 5

# Practicing Ethical Decision-Making

## Adam Burston, Andrew Estefan, and Anthony Tuckett

### INTRODUCTION

Developing, and then utilizing, an ethical framework is a vital resilience resource because it offers a way of thinking through complex or ambiguous problems that do not have easy answers, and which can become a source of stress for nurses. Some people can find the idea of ethics to be slippery and elusive, but for nursing practice, an ethical framework can be essential in guiding nurses to ensure they do no harm and do what is right for both their patients and for the healthcare system more generally.

It is useful to begin by stating that ethics is about what a person ought to do as well as about the kind of person one ought to be and is therefore the highest ideal for humanity to aspire to (Tuckett, 1998). Many people struggle to define ethics precisely, but instead describe what ethics is not. For some, this can make ethics an obscure concept, and ethical conduct a vague or difficult practice. The aim of this chapter is to provide clarity around both the idea and practice of ethics, so that it provides a strong basis for practice. In this way, the confusion, distress, and inertia that can arise in the face of ethical tensions can be dissipated, and what remains is the possibility for positive and expedient critical thinking and intentional actions. Being a critical thinker and being able to act purposefully in order to solve problems are, moreover, two important sources of resilience.

## UNCERTAINTY, TENSION, AND DILEMMAS

Whether they are a registered nurse (RN), advanced nurse practitioner (ANP) or student nurse (SN), nurses make hundreds of decisions in a typical day, which makes nursing work a very heavy cognitive task. But more than that, nurses are required to think about whether their decisions are in the best interest of the patient, will cause the most benefit and bring the least harm, and will also be acceptable to the patient, the family, the community, and the healthcare organization. This requires an ability to think about thinking—a meta-cognitive ability. Chief among the meta-cognitive tasks is the ability to think within an ethical framework. Without such an ethical framework, nurses may lose their way in decision-making, and act automatically, without regard for their context and the unique needs of the patient. Imagine a nurse going from issue to issue, thinking only about the problem, never about the person that it affects.

> *Without an ethical framework, nurses may lose their way in decision-making, and act automatically, without regard for the context and unique needs of the patient.*

Instead we propose that, as a higher ideal, ethics or ethical practice is above the law, but obviously not unlawful; it is above codes of conduct and codes of ethics, though these can guide us and give us strength (Tuckett, 2003). Ethics is also an overarching framework for safe practice.

It is important for nurses to recognize what ethics is and what it is not. To begin, there is a difference among ethical uncertainty, ethical distress, and ethical dilemmas. Uncertainty is where a person may *sense* that something is not right, perhaps because it rests uneasily with their internalized, but unarticulated, values. Distress is when one knows that wrong is occurring and that there is a (perceived) right course of action but constraints prevent this action (Nathaniel, 2006). Finally, there is an ethical dilemma, which is where two opposing but equally right courses of action can be justified. The moral distress often felt in such situations can make nurses feel as if they are being restrained and restricted. There can be numerous constraints to ethical action, including the expectation that nurses will always strictly comply with hospital policy—sometimes even if that policy seems irrelevant or even wrong. There might also be a silencing culture that influences the good nurse to take no action. Such constraints on action can lead to feelings of doubt, anger, exhaustion, low self-esteem, and, finally, surrendering or avoidance behaviors, such as distancing and failure to fully engage with patients' needs or team decisions, and finally, a desire to leave the profession (Burston & Tuckett, 2013). The effects of such distress can be long-lasting. Consider the distress involved in the following story, which is reported from practice.

### Rachel's Story

Rachel (ANP) has worked for over 25 years in oncology and has seen a lot of change including new models of care delivery, changed funding mechanisms, and expansions in the scope of practice for a registered nurse.

Rachel has recently returned from an international conference where she learned about a promising new treatment that would lead to improved practice in her area. Rachel was keen to get the treatment started at her workplace and so approached her clinical supervisor who seemed enthusiastic and explained that the protocol would need to be presented to both the Change Management and Clinical Safety Committees.

Rachel was initially excited, but then learned that this process usually takes around 4 to 6 months. This was a disappointing blow, because she knew that there was plenty of evidence that the treatment led to beneficial outcomes and was, indeed, safer and more economical than what they presently did.

Frustrated, she asked her colleague, "Why does this have to be such a drawn-out process?"

Her colleague shrugged and said, "Just business as usual, I guess."

Despondent, Rachel's thoughts vacillated among "Why should I try and persist with this change? What *must* I do? What *can* I do? *How* can I do it?"

This situation describes the tension that frequently occurs when new knowledge is brought to light that could be utilized to inform and improve practice. Because of the formal structure of hospitals and decision-making processes, delays, impediments, and obstacles to change are common. In addition, a frequent cause of significant distress is working with others not competent to deliver the care required (Burston, Tuckett, Parker, & Eley, 2017). Unmanaged distress in one situation can make a person vulnerable to being easily triggered when another similar situation occurs. As time goes on, unmanaged distress accumulates, leading to disempowerment.

## PREPARING FOR INEVITABLE UNCERTAINTIES AND DILEMMAS

To move beyond the impotence and frustration felt when faced with ethical uncertainty, distress, or dilemmas, it is vital that nurses firstly understand the four principles of ethical practice. These are autonomy, beneficence, nonmaleficence, and justice. These four elements are classically recognized as the principles of bioethics (Beauchamp & Childress, 2009).

> *The four principles of ethics are autonomy, beneficence, nonmaleficence, and justice.*

Autonomy is universally accepted to mean that an individual is self-governing or self-determining (Beauchamp, Walters, Kahn, & Mastroianni, 2014). In other words, autonomy defines a person's capacity to make decisions regarding themselves, free from any coercion from another person. Consequently, in the healthcare environment, great importance is placed on providing patients with information regarding their treatment and treatment options, so that they can make informed decisions about their care. More broadly, respecting autonomy allows individuals the dignity of controlling their own destiny.

Beneficence is concerned with "doing good" and thus the promotion of well-being and quality of life in others (Summers, 2014). A benevolent practitioner will at all times be aware of the patient's situation and facilitate care provision in the *best interest* of that patient (Beauchamp et al., 2014). As such, nurses actively care well by aiming to "do good" at all times.

Nonmaleficence is often set as a companion to the principle of beneficence and is often translated to the idea of "Above all, do no harm" (Kerridge, Lowe, & Stewart, 2013). Nonmaleficence guides nurses to refrain from healthcare decisions and interventions that might harm the patient. This does not, of course, mean that all health interventions are "free of harm" (Summers, 2014), but it does mean that this motivation helps to guide decision-making.

The final principle of justice is more challenging to define since there are numerous ways and theories that can be used to discuss it (Kerridge et al., 2013). Here, and generally speaking, the principle of justice concerns ensuring that all reasonable measures are taken to distribute benefits (and burdens) equally. This is known as "distributive justice" (Beauchamp et al., 2014).

The following story reveals these four principles operating in tension.

## Kwan's Story

When Kwan became a newly Graduated Australian Registered Nurse, he was so joyful because nursing was his dream job. But 2 years after graduating, Kwan is having difficulty adapting to a new rotation, working in a very busy, acute surgical ward.

He began to sense his idealism and self-confidence waver and admitted:, "This is a really hard slog at times. You've got to be careful that the job doesn't creep up on you and bite you! Yeah, I guess I am mostly supported by my colleagues, but boy, I am really tired at times and often wonder if I can keep my head above water. Last evening, for example, I was allocated several postoperative patients, and one more expected to return from theatre. I was barely managing to keep up, when – Pow! – the Nurse Unit Manager told me that one of the other staff had fallen sick and was going home, and wouldn't be replaced for a few hours. I was asked – no, told – to keep an eye on two additional patients until a replacement staff member could be found!"

Thinking about it later, Kwan felt stressed, unsupported, and really doubted himself. He had a whole series of thoughts going through his mind. How can I do this and not make mistakes? How will I manage additional patients when I'm only just managing at the moment? What if the Nurse Unit Manager can't find a replacement? How will I provide the standard of care I am obliged to deliver? What if I don't know enough about the patients to really provide quality care?"

Kwan finds himself grappling with a tension between providing care for an increased number of patients (his workload) and his perceived concern about his level of knowledge and experience to manage these patients (his competence). Kwan's tensions manifest because he lacks the time to provide sufficient care and support to his patients to allow them to make informed decisions (and exercise autonomy). Being time-poor exacerbates Kwan's tensions as he recognizes he is unable to implement the necessary cares that are required (beneficence). Kwan, pushed to practice at the edge of his competence, and although extremely conscious of not wanting to do so, risks "doing harm" (nonmaleficence). Finally, Kwan is only one person where many people are needed to assist in an environment where competing care demands are ongoing. He finds it impossible to ensure that all of his patients have an equal and fair opportunity to access the care that is needed (justice). In addition, as a relatively junior nurse in a very stressful situation, Kwan struggles to make sense of the right thing to do and to communicate his concerns to others.

## Ethical Values

Being able to identify the principles as they occur in the complex reality of practice can be liberating, because nurses can put a name to their sources of frustration. No longer is the stress amorphous and diffuse, as it can be named. Once named, fitting values can be called to mind and then mobilized into action.

Many nursing students choose nursing as a career because they value caring for others. This value is fitting for nursing and should be highly prized and protected. But there are some personal values that do not fit the service of professional nursing, and this is why values are important to reflect on, learn about, and consciously choose to take up as a student moves into the new identity of a professional nurse.

Core ethical values are described in the various codes of ethics for nurses internationally (see, for instance, American Nurses Association [ANA], 2015; International Council of Nurses [ICN],

2012). The ICN *Code of Ethics for Nurses* is premised on four nursing responsibilities. These are the promotion of health, the prevention of illness, the restoration of health, and the alleviation of suffering. These tally with four "principal elements that outline the standards of ethical conduct" (ICN, 2012, p. 2). It is within these four principles that nurses can locate and identify ethical values to think through, manage, and resolve, ethical tensions. These ICN core ethical values are equally represented in the codes of ethics for nurses in other jurisdictions (ANA, 2015) and other disciplines (Australian Medical Association, 2016).

Within the "elements of the code" prescribed by the ICN, RNs, ANPs, and SNs will find the professional ethical values. Equally important and offering guidance, the ICN *Code of Ethics for Nurses* (ICN, 2012) refers to a number of the principles we have previously outlined (Table 5.1).

Notice that the ethical values identified in Table 5.1 make no mention of specific religious or cultural values that may be important personally. Notice, too, that the values stem from acceptance and empathy for the differences of others, and ultimately strive for others to be able to make their own decisions. The overall aim is empowerment. Making conscious use of these nursing values is a source for resilience, and a strategy to empower others.

Table 5.1 Ethical Values and Principles Contained in the International Council of Nurses (2012) *Code of Ethics for Nurses*

| Element of the Code | Ethical Value |
|---|---|
| Nurses and people | Respect for others; respectfulness |
| | Responsiveness |
| | Trustworthiness |
| | Integrity |
| | **Principles** |
| | Autonomy |
| | Confidentiality |
| | Justice (distributive justice) |
| Nurses and coworkers | Beneficence (advocacy) |

*Source:* International Council of Nurses. (2012). *The ICN Code of Ethics for Nurses.* Retrieved from https://www.icn.ch/nursing-policy/regulation-and-education

A next step in clarifying ethics so that it does not remain intangible, but instead becomes a foundation for thinking about patient needs and patient care in a logical and effective way, is to understand the so-called "Golden Rule." The Golden Rule is about standing one's ground, to know what it is that you would want to have happen in a care situation, and to insist on upholding this standard for all others.

## The Golden Rule

Like principles, a rule-based approach to ethical practice or decision-making is action-oriented. Application of the Golden Rule by the nurse answers the question: "How would I want to be treated?" The Golden Rule can be summed up as follows:

> There is a principle which is found and has persisted in many religious and ethical traditions of humankind for thousands of years: What you do not wish done to yourself, do not do to others . . . What you wish done to yourself, do to others. This should be the irrevocable, unconditional norm for all areas of life . . . for families and communities . . . nations. (Küng, 1993, p. 7)

In the *Declaration Toward a Global Ethic*, Hans Küng offers a number of insights about this rule. First, the Golden Rule is universal; that is, it can be affirmed by those who are religious or nonreligious. The emphasis is on its applicability for those seeking *ethical* guidance. Second, the rule is consequentialist in its form (Kerridge et al., 2013); that is, it demands of the RN, APN, or SN to be responsible for her or his "decisions, actions and failures (as having) consequences" (Küng, 1993, p. 6). Third, the rule demands that "every human is obliged to behave in a genuinely human fashion, to do good and avoid evil" (Küng, 1993, p. 7). Last, the guidance offered by the rule posits the client as an end in and of themselves, never a mere means to an end (Küng, 1993).

*Adhere to the Golden Rule—that people should aim to treat each other as they would like to be treated themselves: with tolerance, consideration, and compassion.*

## Ethical Theories

Ethical theories help nursing students understand both the rights and the wrongs of caring; that is, the things to do, and not to do. These rules are reassuring because, if properly applied, ethical reasoning helps nurses to determine defensible actions when caring for others. These rights and wrongs can also create difficulties, however, when the practice situation just does not seem to quite "fit" with certain ethical principles or prevailing practices.

Broadly speaking ethical theories can be descriptive, prescriptive, or applied. Descriptive theories tell us what is happening, prescriptive theories tell us what we ought to do, and applied theories address both of these aspects, usually in a specific context such as nursing. In practice, ethical theories translate into obligations to behave in a certain way. Nurses are required to perform their duties, and ethics provides a framework within which nurses' duties can be understood. The ethics of duty is also referred to as deontology. Deontological theory foregrounds nurses' obligations to safeguard patients' well-being. For example, the practice of monitoring fluid intake and output is a practice that observes, measures, and reports, but it also helps to safeguard the patient from harm, arguably one objective of good nursing care. To not record fluid intake and output represents a failure on the part of the nurse to perform his or her duty.

Deontology, or the ethics of duty, plays an important part in nursing practice. One central component of deontological theory is the notion of reasonableness. That is to say, reasonable people make ethical decisions and act upon them (Kant, 2011). While this is a simplification of a fairly complex ethical theory, it highlights the idea that there has to be a reference point for, or a way to understand, what is considered reasonable nursing behavior in different clinical contexts. For nurses, there are multiple reference points regarding reasonable (and, thus, appropriate and ethical) conduct. For example, education, hospital policy, colleague and interprofessional agreements, and, of course, research that seeks to explore the most efficient and useful ways to care for patients are all points of reference for nurses.

Another group of ethical theories that organizes healthcare practices are the consequentialist theories. Consequentialism, briefly summarized, focuses on outcomes. Whereas deontological theory calls for attention to the right or wrong of a nursing action in terms of duty, consequentialist ethics ties the nursing action to its outcome, result, or effect asking, "Does the outcome justify the action?" Consequentialist ethics seeks a good outcome. Utilitarianism, a form of consequentialist ethics, applies the principle of doing the greatest good for the greatest number. Although in healthcare, we might interpret "good" as being the recovery or reduction of pain, the good that is referred to in foundational utilitarian theory is happiness or pleasure.

Happiness and pleasure are physical and psychosocial phenomena amenable to nursing intervention; for example, implementing nursing measures to reduce pain and discomfort. Importantly, promoting happiness and pleasure for patients goes beyond physical interventions to attending closely to patients' psychosocial dimensions. But how does a busy and sometimes underresourced nurse work adaptively with patients in this way? After all, many healthcare settings are extremely busy and demanding in terms of what nurses have to do. It may be that nurses need to stop and ask "Who are we?" and "How are we?" with patients. Virtue ethics emphasizes precisely this aspect of practice. Virtue ethics begins with the assumption that virtuous or good people make ethical decisions. Virtue ethics is about character, but it is also about what drives or motivates us to care (Greenfield & Banja, 2009). Gordon and Nelson (2006) suggested that nurses have a very strong virtue script, which is reinforced by society. That is to say, nurses, and nursing in general as a profession, are seen as possessing certain characteristics that are important in caring for others. The difficulty this creates for nurses is that these characteristics are viewed as being at odds with other virtues such as being assertive, knowledgeable, independent, and proficient.

As nurses grapple with questions about what to do to care for patients, virtue ethics also calls upon them to consider the sort of nurses they want to be. A consideration of virtue ethics helps nurses to focus on what they do and how they cultivate and enact practice values and behaviors that match with and join together a sense of self as person and self as nurse. In essence, this involves writing a new virtue script: one that claims the ability and capacity to care, but also blends this with personal or self-knowledge and the knowledge and expertise gained from education.

## ADAPTING, CHANGING, AND THINKING ETHICALLY

Nursing can be an extremely fulfilling career. It is a job where no two days are ever the same and a nurse can be sure that they have taken actions to help others. Ideally a nurse will feel each day that they have made a positive difference. But patients' needs are variable and a nurse must have a readiness to adapt, change, and think ethically to meet these needs. Thus, even though a nurse may become so technically competent that the tasks of care are easy, or even routine, the decision-making, fast-pace, and communication challenges persist. Having a process for thinking things through in a reasoned way and then communicating those decisions clearly are sources of resilience and tools to empower self and others.

With resilience strategies, nurses will find a way to learn to deal with ethical issues to improve their practice, rather than be constrained by them. In this section, we share several strategies for doing this, including the development of moral resilience and moral courage, the use of mentors and interprofessional dialogue, and the development of a viable process for ethical decision-making.

### Developing Moral Resilience

Being able to face ethical tensions, process these cognitively, and ultimately cope with the consequences is a vital part of resilience for nurses. Not all of the consequences of ethical reasoning will lead to positive outcomes for patients or staff. Thus, resilience speaks to the ability of the RN, ANP, and SN to manage adversity and "prevail in the face of stress" (Matos, Neushotz, Griffin, & Fitzpatrick, 2010, p. 308). It is important to recognize that how the stress is managed is crucial, not the avoidance of stress and stressful situations, which is impossible in nursing. Rushton (2016) defines moral resilience as "the capacity of an individual to sustain or restore their integrity in response to moral complexity, confusion, distress, or setbacks" (p. 112). Building moral resilience is a way forward in ameliorating the experience of moral distress as a resilient nurse is adept at navigating moral distress. That is, the nurse can not only face the tension (expecting resistance and challenge), but can also expect a positive resolution. This results in a lessening of tension. This is important for developing resilience, as a buildup of moral residue over time exacerbates subsequent experiences of moral distress (Epstein & Hamric, 2009), undermining resilience, exacerbating vulnerability, and risking the longevity of nurses' careers and their health.

## Developing Moral Courage

A particular challenge that often occurs during a situation of moral distress is a sense of powerlessness or helplessness. This is difficult for nurses, because they hold a powerful position in relation to patients and the healthcare system. To suddenly be struck with feelings of impotence and ineffectualness can add to the distress and is understandably difficult. In this moment, it is useful to enact self-compassion, to take some time to wait and think through a course of action, and to seek support. Readers will be familiar with the concept of empathy, having a sense of what another is going through and feeling. Self-compassion is empathy turned inward, toward the self. It is about acknowledging, or being mindful of, one's own suffering or difficulties, to see this as part of maintaining a sense of common humanity, whereby we are all deserving of kindness (Neff, 2016). Equally, it is vital to take a course of action, and not to remain inert or paralyzed, for failing to act can, in itself, be an act of harm (Rodney, 2017). Taking action in the face of moral distress, despite fear or other anxiety, constitutes moral courage (Dolan, 2016). Moral courage is what is needed among healthcare colleagues and in healthcare services. It is both an act/series of actions, and an attitude, that builds personal resilience, the resilience of patients, and the resilience and purpose of healthcare organizations.

## Mentorship

Mentorship is another important strategy that facilitates the continued development of (moral) resilience by targeting the issues underlying and causing moral distress, working through them in supportive relationships (Musto, Rodney, & Vanderheide, 2014). Ideally, mentorship provides an opportunity for the mentor to challenge the mentee to explore his or her own thoughts, feelings, and values, and to enact self-regulation by using such proven strategies as self-calming, self-validation, and self-kindness (Rushton, 2016).

To be effective, mentoring is not a one-off meeting instituted at the time of an ethical issue, but should be a relationship that is developed, cultivated, and exercised over time. Therefore, healthcare organizations need to see the benefits of mentorship and formally support mentorship relationships that are focused on the exploration of difficult issues and ways of using the tools of self-compassion. Active measures to initiate mentorships include instituting a policy of assigning an ethical practice/decision-making mentor to new staff and introducing a mechanism to support new mentorship arrangements in circumstances where the initial arrangement is not working, unproductive, or the mentor leaves the organization.

The knowledge, experience, and skills of the ethical practice/decision-making mentor are crucial to the effectiveness and efficacy of the mentorship experience. The mentor must be clinically experienced, have demonstrated reasoned decision-making over a considerable time period, and have voluntarily agreed to undertake the ethical practice/decision-making mentor role. We also recommend that this person resides elsewhere within the organization and is not likely to be directly exposed to the specific ethical tensions faced by the mentee. Lastly, the mentor must be able to create a safe space for ethically focused discourse to occur without retribution. The mentor must be able to guide the mentee in unpacking complex ethical tensions, challenge the mentee's ethical beliefs, and support the mentee in developing an increased level of moral courage. This safe place should be available on a regular (ideally at least monthly) basis, as well as ad hoc (when required).

## Interprofessional Dialogue

Ethical issues in healthcare frequently involve multiple professionals from various disciplines. As a result, the uncertainty, distress, and tensions that arise because of such ethical dilemmas can negatively affect many people. Therefore, it is important to maintain open, honest and supportive dialogue among the multidisciplinary team (Lachman, 2016) and to allow disciplinary differences to be aired. There are many strategies that can be used to put this dialogue into operation. Informal clinical ward conversations are one strategy, and interprofessional ethics education a more formal option.

The informal process has the benefit of being accessible, and at the bedside, which allows nurses to readily engage with colleagues such as doctors and physiotherapists about real-world ethical tensions as they are unfolding, or soon after they are exposed. This interaction can take place at the clinical interface with the patient and the attending healthcare providers, becoming a naturally occurring interaction. This process requires courage to speak up about problems and concerns and is contingent on the previously recommended strategies of self-compassion and having instituted supportive mentor relationships. Holding such conversations is useful however, because it may relieve pent up distress, clarify feelings into thoughts, and assist the group in cultivating an honest, open, and healthy workplace.

The formal process generally involves a series of facilitated formal workshops led by a clinical ethicist. Here the nurse and other healthcare workers learn about clinical ethics and are given opportunities to openly discuss its application in their clinical contexts and air their experiences in cognate areas.

Formal processes occur in many major health services and university organizations and is a forum for interprofessional discussion of contemporary ethical tensions. Generally, a case study is presented and discussion is facilitated by a professional clinical ethicist. The goal is to examine ethical tensions and cultivate shared understandings as well as acknowledging differences among the professions and, at times, how individuals from these professions may approach ethical issues in varying ways.

## A Process for Ethical Decision-Making

A decision-making framework is an important cognitive tool that simplifies complexity (Figure 5.1). In emotionally charged and complex clinical situations, it may not be easy to think issues through clearly. Without clear thinking on ethical dilemmas, nurses may give up on the challenging work of participating in the decision-making process. Nonparticipation is not a choice, however, because being a bystander to breaches of trust, unfairness, or wrong-doing is being complicit and adding to the harm of patients. Therefore, being able to recall this framework and implement the steps to assist patient safety, well-being, and quality of life will be an empowering strategy for you.

The first step when you encounter a difficult situation is to clarify the problem. This requires that you assemble your thoughts, values, and biases, and the thoughts, values, and needs of the stakeholders. It requires moral courage to admit concerns, and is a good time to access a mentor to assist you to reason through the issue. Call to mind

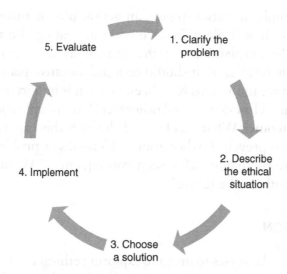

**Figure 5.1** Ethical decision-making framework.
*Source:* Winnipeg Regional Health Authority. (2015). *Ethical decision-making framework: Evidence informed practice tool*. Retrieved from http://www.mb-phen.ca/files/EthicsEIPT.pdf

the professional code of ethics at this stage. Ask yourself, what type of person am I to be? Activate empathy and listen deeply so that you can actually identify the values and needs of others in this situation. What worries you? Are there competing interests?

The second step is to describe the problem in terms of ethical theory. Here interprofessional dialogue will be useful. Perhaps you can contact the health-service ethicist, or a university ethics committee secretary for advice. This requires you to draw upon utilitarian, deontological, relational, or virtue ethics. List the ethical principles involved. Recall the principles of autonomy, beneficence, nonmaleficence, and justice so that you appreciate what or whether a breach is occurring. Write down the ethical problem, stating all facts and preferences. For example, if an issue of harm to the patient is occurring, it is a breach of beneficence, and so on.

The next step is to brainstorm solutions and gradually reduce the options by eliminating those that are not acceptable to the stakeholders. The choice made needs to be something that people can act on, logistically and morally. It may not be unanimous, but everyone should be able to understand the rationale and be able to live with the decision. Here it is important to gain support from the team either through the informal process of a clinical ward conversation or through the formal institutional ethical process.

In the implementation phase, an action plan is made and put into practice. It will likely involve communicating the actions to all stakeholders, explaining why the decision has been made and its intended benefits; that is, it should be a collaborative plan of action.

Finally, after the actions have been taken, it is important to evaluate the impact. How do you and others feel? Are people comfortable with the outcome? What was learned through this experience that can be used to prevent further ethical dilemmas or problems in the future? Were there any unforeseen consequences? What could be done differently in the future?

## CONCLUSION

This chapter asks nurses to imagine exploring ethical tensions in their clinical practice. Unresolved ethical tensions have the capacity to cause harm to all those involved, and especially to the nurse. If the nursing profession is to flourish, then individual nurses need to be resilient—and one important mechanism to facilitate this is to develop an ethical framework for practice, and then mobilize this in difficult situations. If so, ethical tensions, as insistent and often difficult to process as they can be in healthcare, will then cease to be overwhelming or impossible to resolve for the individual nurse. Knowing how to act in ambiguous situations is freeing for both the nurse and his or her patients.

Ethical practice is the highest ideal needed for humanity to flourish and is concerned with what we *ought* to do (how nurses act) as well as the kind of person we *ought* to be (how nurses are). Nurses must, therefore, strive for this ideal whenever they encounter ethical tensions in the workplace. The effects of unresolved tensions manifest as moral distress, which is detrimental to both the individual nurse and the nursing workforce. Instead, ethical practice is achievable through undertaking strategies aimed at building resilience and moral courage in both individual nurses and groups of nurses in the workplace.

### LEARNING ACTIVITIES

1. Going back to Rachel's story, identify and explain whether Rachel is experiencing uncertainty, distress, or a dilemma. And consider these prompts to help you elaborate on your answer.

- Why do you think Rachel feels this way?
- How may the effects of moral distress impact on Rachel's capacity to function in her day-to-day work?
- In what ways may the effects of this distress impact on the patient experience and, on the culture of the working environment (both short and long term)?

2. Facilitate a group discussion on the following:
   What is competence? How it is demonstrated? And how does it change day to day? Begin the discussion with competence in a general sense, and then focus specifically on ethical competence.

3. Reflect on the four principles of ethics and the questions Kwan asks himself. Are any of the four principles at risk of being compromised?

4. Discuss among your colleagues their understanding of the *Code of Ethics for Nurses* in your jurisdiction. What working knowledge do they have of it? How do they understand how the code is to be used?

5. Compare your personal values with the ethical values that define your profession. How do they match up? Do you think you could work as a nurse if your values were discordant with those of your profession? What challenges may emanate from this discordance?

6. Consider a situation from your own clinical practice where you have grappled with a tension between best practice and the current implementation of care.
   - Reflect on the factors contributing to the situation, the impact on yourself and on the patient(s) involved.
   - Identify the ethical basis of your distress in that situation.
   - Identify strategies you used to manage this distress.
   - If you believe your distress was not managed well, hypothesize strategies that could have been used to improve the experience
   - Explain how you have changed or could change your practice as a result.

7. Discuss the following:
   - Consequentialism (utilitarianism) is an ethical theory. What is its premise?
   - Deontology is an ethical theory. Who is its "famous" proponent and what did he say about how we should treat one another?

**8.** Discuss the following from the nurse's and the patient's perspectives and what this means for daily nursing practice: "I would want to be included in the process of my care; I want to know what is happening and what has happened as it relates to my treatments; I would want to have input into the future of my well-being; I would want my personal and cultural biographies understood and appreciated; I would want truthfulness and to be treated with respect and dignity at all times."

## REFERENCES

American Nurses Association. (2015). *Code of ethics with interpretative statements.* Retrieved from https://www.nursingworld.org/practice-policy/nursing-excellence/ethics/code-of-ethics-for-nurses

Australian Medical Association. (2016). *AMA Code of Ethics 2004. Editorially Revised 2006. Revised 2016.* Retrieved from https://ama.com.au/media/new-code-ethics-doctors

Beauchamp, T., & Childress, J. (2009). *Principles of biomedical ethics* (6th ed.). Oxford, UK: Oxford University Press.

Beauchamp, T., Walters, L., Kahn, J., & Mastroianni, A. (2014). *Contemporary issues in bioethics* (8th ed.). Boston, MA: Wadsworth Cengage.

Burston, A., & Tuckett, A. (2013). Moral distress in nursing: Contributing factors, outcomes and interventions. *Nursing Ethics, 20*(3), 312–324. doi:10.1177/0969733012462049

Burston, A., Tuckett, A., Parker, D., & Eley, R. (2017). Validation of an instrument to measure moral distress within the Australian residential and community care environments. *International Journal of Older People Nursing, 12(2)*, 1–10. doi:10.1111/opn.12139

Dolan, C. (2016). Moral, ethical, and legal decision-making in controversial practice situations. *The Journal for Nurse Practitioners, 13*(2), e57–e65. doi:10.1016/j.nurpra.2016.10.017

Epstein, E. G., & Hamric, A. B. (2009). Moral distress, moral residue, and the crescendo effect. *The Journal of Clinical Ethics, 20*(4), 330–342.

Gordon, S., & Nelson, S. (2006). Moving beyond the virtue script in nursing: Creating a knowledge-based identity for nurses. In S. Nelson & S. Gordon (Eds.), *Complexities of care: Nursing reconsidered* (pp. 13–29). London, UK: ILR Press.

Greenfield, B., & Banja, J. (2009). The role of ethical theory in ethical education for physical therapist students. *Journal of Physical Therapy Education, 23*(2), 24–28. doi:10.1097/00001416-200907000-00004

International Council of Nurses. (2012). *The ICN Code of Ethics for Nurses.* Retrieved from https://www.icn.ch/nursing-policy/regulation-and-education

Kant, I. (2011). *Groundwork of the metaphysics of morals: A German–English edition* (M. Gregor & J. Timmermann, Ed. and Trans.). Cambridge, UK: Cambridge University Press.

Kerridge, I., Lowe, M., & Stewart, C. (2013). *Ethics and law for the health professions* (4th ed.). Annandale, NSW, Australia: Federation Press.

Küng, H. (1993). *Declaration toward a global ethic.* Paper presented at the Council for a Parliament of the World's Religions, Chicago.

Lachman, V. D. (2016). Moral resilience: Managing and preventing moral distress and moral residue. *MEDSURG Nursing, 25*(2), 121-124.

Matos, P. S., Neushotz, L. A., Griffin, M. T. Q., & Fitzpatrick, J. J. (2010). An exploratory study of resilience and job satisfaction among psychiatric nurses working in inpatient units. *International Journal of Mental Health Nursing, 19*(5), 307–312. doi:10.1111/j.1447-0349.2010.00690.x

Musto, L., Rodney, P., & Vanderheide, R. (2014). Toward interventions to address moral distress: Navigating structure and agency. *Nursing Ethics, 22,* 91–102. doi:10.1177/0969733014534879

Nathaniel, A. K. (2006). Moral reckoning in nursing. *Western Journal of Nursing Research, 28*(4), 419–438. doi:10.1177/0193945905284727

Neff, K. D. (2016). Self-compassion. In I. Ivtzan & T. Lomas (Eds.), *Mindfulness in positive psychology: The science of meditation and wellbeing* (pp. 37–50). London, UK: Routledge.

Rodney, P. (2017). What we know about moral distress. *AJN, American Journal of Nursing, 117*(2, Suppl. 1), S7–S10. doi:10.1097/01.NAJ.0000512204.85973.04

Rushton, C. H. (2016). Moral resilience: A capacity for navigating moral distress in critical care. *AACN Advanced Critical Care, 27*(1), 111–119. doi:10.4037/aacnacc2016275

Summers, J. (2014). Principles of healthcare ethics. In E. E. Morrison & B. Furlong (Eds.), *Health care ethics: Critical issues for the 21st century* (pp. 47–63). Burlington, MA: Jones & Bartlett.

Tuckett, A. (1998). An ethic of the fitting: A conceptual framework for nursing practice. *Nursing Inquiry, 5*(4), 220–227. doi:10.1046/j.1440-1800.1998.00241.x

Tuckett, A. (2003). An ethic of fitting: A conceptual framework for nursing practice. In S. Zinaich & J. Rowan (Eds.), *Ethics for the professions* (pp. 278–282). Wadsworth, OH: Belmont.

Winnipeg Regional Health Authority. (2015). *Ethical decision-making framework: Evidence informed practice tool.* Retrieved from http://www.mb-phen.ca/files/EthicsEIPT.pdf

# 6

# Appraising and Moderating Stressful Situations

Rachael R. Sharman, Julie Hanson, and Mary Katsikitis

## INTRODUCTION

Everyone encounters stressful situations in their daily work life. But how does the way these situations are perceived (or thought about) and understood, affect our reactions to them? Success in any profession requires an ability to make clear judgments and to moderate "natural" responses to a stressful encounter. In this chapter, we discuss the influence of appraisals—the judgments we make—during a stressful scenario and how these appraisals might affect our reactions under stress. We will compare the impact of different appraisal and reactive styles on work performance and functioning, particularly in terms of how perceptions and judgments affect both nurses and those around them. Two stories, "First day nerves" and "Constant demands," illustrate the processes that can be used to identify and modify patterns of thinking using psychological approaches. Some tips on how to moderate reactions under stress to make clearer and more widely beneficial professional judgments are also provided.

## FIRST DAY NERVES

It is nursing student Robbie's first day on a new rotation. She is nervous because she has heard rumors that the ward she has been allocated is "difficult" to work in. Robbie is eager to make a good first impression, but the day does not start well. She has difficulty finding a parking space—she did not expect that the staff parking at the hospital would be so crowded and expensive. As she rushes to the ward, she quickly became lost in the labyrinth of corridors and realized that she will be lucky to arrive on time. Feeling pressured and frustrated, Robbie could feel her heart racing. She arrives and introduces herself to the nurse unit manager with apologies for her lateness but is immediately relieved when the manager sympathizes with the parking issues and Robbie's difficulty in finding the ward. The manager then offers to show Robbie around and introduces her to the staff on the ward. Most of the staff members seem friendly and pleasant. Although a little preoccupied with their tasks at hand, they briefly stop to smile, shake Robbie's hand, and welcome her to the ward. Robbie starts to relax a little and begins to look forward to the day ahead.

Suddenly, a physician strides quickly into the area. The physician looks angry. A few orders are briskly directed at another nurse across the other side of the room, about a patient in Room 3. The physician leans over the main counter, snatches a medical file, and proceeds to read it intently.

Robbie stands there, saying nothing, not knowing what to do, and notices her heart has begun to beat quickly again.

Suddenly, the physician looks up, notices Robbie, turns to the unit manager, and asks, "Who's this?"

The manager politely introduces the physician as the "doctor in charge" and introduces Robbie as the new nursing student. Unlike everyone else, the physician makes no move to acknowledge Robbie at all, just looks back at the medical file in his hand, sighs and says, "Oh, fantastic!"

It is illuminating to consider how *you* think Robbie feels about this encounter and how *you* interpret the physician's behavior and comment. Do you think the physician is pleased to have Robbie on the ward that day, or was the new nurse just another nuisance in the already hectic schedule? What do you think Robbie's immediate response would be to this situation? Would she be thrilled that the physician has given a sigh of relief and that her presence here was "fantastic"? Should the nurse sympathize with the physician for having a bad day? Or should the nurse interpret the sigh and comment as a sarcastic gesture? If so, should she shrug off the remark, or, should she have a rising feeling of dread about the new job?

It is important to recognize that each individual's interpretation and reaction to this situation may have more to do with their current physiological state and inbuilt personal thinking styles, rather than an objective analysis of what had occurred. Any of the reactions listed may be considered—by different people—to be totally justified under the circumstances. How each of us thinks and feels about any situation is a highly individual process. However, each of the preceding different reactive styles can be taken to their logical conclusions to assess the impact they will have on both nurses and the people around them.

## THE FUNCTIONAL IMPACT OF REACTIVE STYLES

*How you interpret situations may have more to do with your personal thinking styles than the event itself.*

An important thing to consider is how would each of these very different reactions mentioned earlier affect both a nurse's work performance and functioning and the functioning of the people around the nurse? The following analyses the *functional impact* of each reactive style.

1. The nurse is thrilled that the doctor has indicated that her presence on the ward is "fantastic!" Some readers will be surprised to read this—disbelieving that anyone would have interpreted the situation in this way. There are, however, individuals who have what psychologists call an *optimistic explanatory style* (Peterson, 2000). Like any reactive style, it has its strengths and weaknesses (Tennen & Affleck, 1987). These are the people who happily take credit for their successes but minimize their personal involvement in any failures. They

tend to filter information in a very self-protective manner, ignoring negative feedback and maximizing positive feedback (Lazarus, 1983; Martin-Krumm, Sarrazin, Peterson, & Famose, 2003). Before assuming that such people are all delusional or narcissistic (and it is no surprise, but this style is highly correlated with both), in most (mild-to-moderate) cases, this style makes for a fairly, functional person (Martin-Krumm et al., 2003; Taylor & Brown, 1988). These people interpret everything in the most positive light possible and are almost impossible to offend. They may be viewed by colleagues as unrealistic due to their overly optimistic response to abso-lutely everything, or perhaps even a bit "full of themselves." However, their confidence, sunny dispositions, and thick hides make them enjoyable and often fun to have around. The major downside to individuals with this reactive style is that they can be insensitive to the needs, or state, of those around them. This person may be the one who responds to the physician's comment by slapping them on the back and saying, "That's great. I'm very glad to be here!" The nurse may then try to engage the physician in further conversa-tion, despite it being obvious that he has other pressing things on his mind. In this response, the nurse is not trying to be sarcastic or funny; such personalities just assume that everyone thinks well of them. The downside is that they can, therefore, be insensitive to the negative signals coming from others and react inappropriately at times.

2. The nurse sympathizes with the physician and assumes he is having a bad day. This kind of reaction is known as an *external attribution* toward the physician. The focus is taken off the nurse in question and placed squarely back on the doctor. People who react in this way interpret this situation as being largely about the physician's situation. Hence, they are likely to feel empathy and compassion for the physician's needs, rather than take offense that their own needs, or feelings, have been violated in any way. In this way, they also deflect any negative self-view and, in doing so, often project a kindness toward others that is usually noticed and well received. People who react in this manner may be said to "rise above the situation" and, again, are usually valued as thoughtful and kind employees in the

workplace. Happily, they also do not suffer negative emotion toward themselves—after all, it is the physician who is having the bad day, not them.

3. The nurse interprets the physician's remark as sarcastic but shrugs it off. In this case, the nurse has made an *internal attribution* toward the physician's motives—perhaps, he is a bad-tempered person or has no manners. On the face of it, this seems like a fairly functional response. But even if the nurse casually shrugs off the comment, she has still interpreted some level of malice in the physician's response to her. People who react in this way may, in the future, feel some distaste or dislike for, and even avoid, this physician. They may engage in giving the physician the silent treatment or use a terse manner toward them until they receive an apology. Their thinking at this moment may take the following form: "The physician is being sarcastic; the physician is rude; the physician is being horrible to me and I have done nothing to deserve this, but I am just going to ignore it because the physician is just arrogant." So, while the immediate effect on those around the nurse is neutral (as the nurse does not obviously respond one way or the other), the functional impact of this response on *the nurse* is likely to be negative. This negative impact may then continue to influence how that nurse deals with the other person in the future and is likely to harbor some malice toward him.

4. Tears well up and the nurse feels a rising wave of dread about the new job. This reactive style is probably the most dysfunctional, both for the nurse and the people around her. However, this style is very common, especially among younger people who tend to be a lot more self-conscious and certainly less experienced at processing what other people think of them. People with this reactive style interpret the event as being all about them, rather than being about the physician's manner or their current circumstances. Psychologists call this a *pessimistic explanatory style* (Dykema, Bergbower, & Peterson, 1995) and, over time, people with this reactive style tend to have impaired job performance and experience more physical illness and more social distress (Jackson, Sellers, & Peterson, 2002; Peterson, Seligman, & Vaillant, 1988). It is also important to consider that when the nurse feels distressed and offended, and others

see the tears welling in her eyes, they may feel upset for her. The unit manager may initially react with surprise but will then try to reassure the new nurse. The physician may apologize, but he may also become irritated by the nurse's reaction. If the physician's comment was meant kindly, he may even take offense at the nurse's reaction. Any way this reaction is looked at, the functional impact of this behavior is to take everyone's focus off his or her job at that moment and place it squarely onto the nurse. For obvious reasons, this reactive style is the one least valued in workplaces. Work colleagues learn they have to worry about that individual's reactions, feel they are "walking on egg shells" and need to take valuable time out of their hectic schedules to deal with another's emotions. Furthermore, and worst of all, *that nurse* also feels awful—so this is very much a lose–lose situation for everyone involved.

### Evaluating and Moderating Your Reactive Style

When you find yourself feeling, thinking, and reacting in a particular way, ask yourself these questions:

- What purpose does this reaction serve?
- How does this reaction make me feel?
- How does it affect my functioning?
- What are the likely effects (both positive and negative) of this reaction on those around me?

Try to think of the functional effects of your reaction and, in essence, what will be achieved by reacting this way.

If everyone could moderate emotions easily and shift reactions to this-or-that style, there would be none of the wonderful variety in human interaction that makes daily life so rich and interesting. As a result, we are not suggesting that an individual can (or should) always fully control his or her natural reactive style, but we are saying that each nurse should at least be prepared to do a double take, to reassess and to re-evaluate how he or she is interpreting and responding to the environment. You may be surprised to find there are ways of changing your perceptions and reactive style, which will also change the way you feel and cope. We discuss these in the next section.

*The way we perceive and respond to other people is a highly individual trait, usually operating on a continuum from optimistic to pessimistic. Before you react, think about the functional implications of your reaction and ask yourself: How will my response affect me and the people around me? Will my reaction hinder or help?*

## LEARNING TO CHANGE YOUR REACTIVE STYLE

### The Impact of Physiological Arousal

Have you ever misinterpreted a situation when you were angry? Perhaps, you have interpreted a harmless comment as a threat or an insult. Conversely, have you ever felt wildly attracted to someone during a highly emotional situation? This could be, for example, while on holidays, during a stressful work or university project, or while on the rebound from a relationship.

Not everyone knows that their current state of physiological arousal can affect their perceptions of the surrounding environment and their subsequent emotional response. In 1974, Dutton and Aron conducted an important experiment, often referred to as the "rickety bridge" test. Young men crossed one of two bridges, one of which was "rickety" and looked dangerous, to meet an attractive female research assistant, who in turn asked each one a series of questions. The psychologists were interested in whether the high physiological arousal created in the men who crossed the dangerous looking bridge—and had their heart and respiratory rates and adrenaline levels thus raised—could then be (mis)attributed by the men as a feeling of desire, or even lust, for the attractive woman. The experiment found that the effect of high physiological arousal on the men's reactions to the research assistant was electrifying. Four times as many men who crossed the rickety bridge, compared with those who crossed another safer bridge, subsequently made contact with the research assistant to ask her to go out on a date.

Experiments like this are often cited as evidence that individuals can misattribute their current level of physiological arousal to factors in the environment (Pham, 2007; White, Fishbein, & Rutsein, 1981). These men only differed in whether their heart and respiratory rates and adrenaline were elevated when they met the research assistant. The high-arousal group assumed that she was the cause of this feeling and therefore interpreted their physiological arousal as being caused by the attractiveness of the female assistant, when it was actually caused by their crossing of the bridge. Such misattribution can, of course, lead to several errors.

Robbie, the apprehensive student nurse at the beginning of this chapter was stressed by her late arrival and the crowded and expensive car park and her frustration with getting lost. Her heart rate was raised, she was feeling flustered and her physiology was on high alert. The rickety bridge experiment suggests that this would obviously have affected her interpretation of the physician's comment. Previous research suggests that people in this high-arousal state are much more likely to become defensive or upset, which is manifested as anger and distress (Rule & Nesdale, 1976; Wild, Clark, Ehlers, & McManus, 2006). Human beings are concerned with cause and effect; in other words, if a nurse feels stressed, the nurse wants to know what caused it. If a hapless physician marches into the immediate environment and makes an ambiguous comment—then, the physician must be the cause of how the nurse is feeling. Just like the men who misattributed their high level of arousal to the female research assistant, it is alarmingly easy for anyone to make the same error.

*Next time you are on "high alert," with your adrenaline racing, be aware that your interpretations of subsequent situations may be colored by this high-arousal state.*

It is common to warn people not to make a decision while their "blood is boiling" or to counsel them to "keep a cool head" under pressure. This advice is supported by research that indicates decision-making is impaired when physiological arousal is high enough to be stressful (Wild et al., 2006). Keinan (1987) found that this impairment mostly resulted from people not assessing all available information; essentially, jumping to conclusions. In contrast, a moderate level of physiological arousal promotes productive decision-making, functioning, and "rising to the challenge" (Seo & Barrett, 2007). But once the level of physiological arousal gets too high, the brain can interpret the situation as stressful, and anything in the immediate environment can mistakenly be attributed as causing, or contributing to, that stress.

Health professionals working in hospital settings need to be especially mindful of this effect because they are working in an environment in which many heart-racing moments abound. Anesthetists, for example, are known to describe their jobs as "99% pure boredom and 1% pure terror," in reference to the usually routine nature of their work, coupled with the rare, but potentially fatal, complications of anesthesia. Emergency nurses, midwives, and surgery nurses are all guaranteed some heart-stopping, and heart-starting, moments. In such instances, their interpretation of events will be affected.

How might you perceive the interactions with your patients and their caregivers when you are in a stressful situation? In thinking about this, you also need to consider how others in that high state of physiological arousal might interpret your actions? Be prepared for unrealistic accusations, threats, and insults to be directed at you when others make erroneous decisions while they are stressed and their "blood is boiling." This may particularly be the case with patients who are undergoing a frightening, or even life-threatening, procedure.

So what should nurses do in such a situation? First, they should be aware of their current level of arousal and be mindful that this can, and does, affect interpretation of what's going on around them. When in a state of high arousal, an individual is predisposed to misinterpret events or comments as threatening or insulting and can, in response, react defensively. Sometimes, the best advice in this situation is the oldest: Breathe deeply and count to 10 slowly, before making any response. This suggestion has stood the test of time because it is a relaxation technique that lowers arousal and, in doing so, allows the person to reappraise their situation with a "cool head." Reactions made in anger and defense can be hard to erase from others' memories and, even worse, can escalate an ordinary situation into a bad one, and a bad situation into a catastrophe.

In trying to appraise what is going on when you feel stressed, ensure that you are in as relaxed state as possible; this strategy will substantially minimize the potentially disastrous errors of poor judgment that commonly occur in these circumstances. If on the receiving end of someone else's misattribution or misinterpretation, it is important to not respond defensively. Instead, calmly restate your position, perhaps giving the other person an opportunity to retreat with dignity. A comment like, "Oh, I'm sorry, I am not being clear. What I mean is ... " is useful in such a situation as it allows the addition of clarification and explanation.

> *Reactions made in anger can be hard to erase from the memories of those around you.*

Any technique that can be used to relax and return the physiology to normal can be used in such situations. It is important that, rather than responding in anger, to, if necessary, debrief *after* any event in which offense could be taken. Taking a well-considered approach is much more functional than reacting, possibly mistakenly, in a highly emotional moment.

> *When you are at a stressful level of physiological arousal, you are prone to errors in decision-making and defensive reactions. Realize that you and your patients are prone to misinterpreting each others' reactions as threatening or insulting during periods of high physiological arousal. Before responding here, try to calm yourself down or calm your patient down.*

## Appraisals and Judgments: Changing Reactions

You are tucked up warm in bed on a rainy night. Suddenly, from your comfy bed, you hear a loud bang. You jerk into alertness, your heart races, and your breathing quickens. But how do you interpret the bump in the night? And how does that affect the way you react? If you assume that it is the sound of the cat jumping off the couch, you will most likely roll over and go straight back to sleep. But what if you interpret the bump as a recently escaped criminal trying to get in? Now, how do you feel? Now you are certainly not inclined to roll over and go back to sleep. Instead, your heart rate escalates, your adrenaline starts pumping, and you are preparing to flee or fight. This is because you appraised the bump in the night as danger. In reality, both reactions are equally as unfounded. In the absence of getting out of bed and checking, there is no real evidence to suggest what caused the noise and what level of reaction is valid.

The effect of how a particular event is appraised, or thought about, can markedly alter the interpretation of that event and the reaction to it. To go back to the nurse in the story at the beginning of this chapter, there were four very different appraisals proposed, and each elicited a very different reaction:

1. The nurse takes the physician at face value, appraises the behavior as welcoming, and takes the comment as a compliment.
2. The nurse appraises the physician as having a bad day and therefore does not take the comment personally.
3. The nurse appraises a level of sarcasm in the physician's sigh and comment, and so does take it personally, but moves on.
4. The nurse appraises the physician's comment as insulting and offensive, takes it personally, and reacts with distress.

The key to moderating reactions in stressful situations is to attempt to reappraise what has happened. The particular importance of this approach if your own physiological level of arousal is high or at stressful levels has been discussed. Now, we will outline the simple steps that can be taken to reappraise a situation if you feel you are about to react in a dysfunctional manner (such as with anger or distress).

1. Take stock of your own physiology. Are you in a high arousal or stressed state? If so, do nothing in the moment. Instead, leave any response until later, when you have had a chance to reappraise the situation in a calm and relaxed state. Your likelihood of making an accurate judgment and responding in a functional manner will then be greatly increased.
2. Return again to the nurse–physician interaction outlined earlier. What was your first impression as you read that story? Which response do you think you would most likely have made? Your next step is to generate as many other "possible appraisals" as you can. The physician has made an ambiguous statement, so what are some other ways you could think about the intent or meaning of that statement? You can then practice this technique in a range of settings.

3. Seek feedback from others. If, after a calm reappraisal of the evidence, you are still certain that a work colleague or patient is being rude or unreasonable, check with others about their appraisal of the situation. Have you ever said to someone, "Hey, what's wrong with him? Doesn't he like me or something?" Then you are told that the person in question is in terrible circumstances at present, or is battling a health condition, or that he is like that toward everyone, so not to take it personally. This advice can help you to reappraise the scenario and to respond more functionally.

4. If, and only if, it is agreed in a calm and considered manner that someone has, in fact, been unreasonable toward you, then the next steps need to be considered carefully. Again, consider the effects of the fourth appraisal and reaction described earlier. In other words, no matter how justified you may be in becoming upset, it is not going to help. At this point, consultation with your supervisor may be necessary. Then you can put forth, in as calm and objective a manner as possible, what happened, what your reaction was, and what you think needs to change to help you function better in the environment or situation in future.

To return to the example of nurse Robbie and what steps would make for a functional response in this situation: The situation presents itself such that the physician makes an ambiguous comment while the nurse was in a flustered state. These steps can be followed for a resolution that all involved can live with.

1. The nurse should acknowledge she is in a high-arousal state and say nothing in the moment. They should wait until their physiology has returned to normal to think through the issues.

2. Once the nurse has a "cool head," she should generate as many reappraisals as possible in order to explain the physician's response. The nurse should then assess which one seems most reasonable or most likely.

3. If the nurse is still concerned that what has occurred is unreasonable, the nurse should seek opinions from others about how she perceived the situation. This needs to be done in the most discreet manner possible to avoid being accused of being a gossip or troublemaker. As the nurse is new, the most appropriate person from whom to seek advice would be the nurse unit manager.

4. The nurse needs to take ownership of her personal reactions. In seeking advice, she should calmly put forth what happened and be very specific about what she found offensive, and why. For example, the following explanation could be a specific summary of Robbie's thoughts and feelings: "I got really upset when the physician said that. It was my first day. I was nervous, everyone else was being really nice and I thought what the physician said was rude."

5. If people agree that what happened was unreasonable, the nurse should take it to a supervisor for further discussion. It is up to each nurse to resolve such situations, and supervisors, having worked in the setting for much longer, will be in a better position to judge how best to handle the situation.

*How we feel about a situation is closely linked to how we appraise what has just happened. Before reacting, consider other possible appraisals; if necessary, seek input from others as to how they appraised the situation. If you are still upset, seek advice from your supervisor.*

## CONSTANT DEMANDS

The following story illustrates a more complex scenario, one in which the misattributions appear to be coming from a patient's reading of the events when feeling stressed and vulnerable. The story demonstrates the impact that a potential human error of judgment can make on a patient's recovery.

Melanie is an experienced nurse. She has worked on medical and surgical wards for several years and is proficient in caring for highly dependent patients. On arrival for a night shift, Melanie is allocated one of the high dependency bays on the medical ward. She has three patients, one of whom, a middle-aged man, had been transferred from the cardiothoracic intensive care unit that evening, following triple by-pass surgery the previous morning. She has mapped out a mental plan of the three patients' care needs and begins the shift by introducing herself to the patients. Melanie prioritizes an elderly woman who had a heart catheterization procedure earlier that day and whose wound site is due to be checked.

The middle-aged man calls Melanie over to his bedside. He asks her to change the television channel for him because he does not have a remote control and she can see that he cannot easily lean forward and reach the control panel because of his chest wound. Melanie readily assists him and finds the sports channel for him and he seems content with that. She then returns to the elderly patient. However, the middle-aged man calls her once more. He is not happy with the sports channel—he has already watched the game that is being broadcast and he wants "his" nurse to find something more interesting for him. Melanie goes over to him, suggests a news channel as his next option and he nods in agreement. Once this is set, she again returns to her observations of the elderly woman. Within a few minutes, the middle-aged man shouts over to Melanie again. As Melanie approaches, she notices that he looks restless, uncomfortable, and sweaty. His heart monitor shows an increasing heart rate and Melanie interprets this as a sign that his condition is unstable. He demands that she change the television channel again but Melanie is more concerned with his current signs and symptoms and gently asks if he has any chest pain or discomfort. He confirms that he has chest pain. The hospital chest pain protocol requires that Melanie completes a set of observations and performs an EKG. Melanie quickly assembles the equipment at the man's bedside but he will not answer any questions about his pain score, pushes her hand away as they try to take his blood pressure and, when the nurse starts to explain the need for an EKG, is adamant that he does not need a recording. He scowls at Melanie and starts speaking loudly enough to attract the attention of other staff members and patients.

"There is nothing wrong with my heart. It is you. You're the problem. You cannot even change the TV channel for me, so how can you expect me to relax and trust you to look after me properly tonight? I want another nurse, not you. Someone capable!"

In this case, the patient is making some attributions, which are likely affecting his response. It is worth asking about his current physiology and his mood state. The nurse needs to ask how he is reacting or "acting these out," and how does his reaction affect her job. What could a nurse do to calm the patient, and to offer the best possible healthcare in this situation?

It is important in these circumstances to remember that the patient, simply by virtue of having invasive and life-changing surgery, is already in a high state of arousal and is, most likely, experiencing an equally high level of anxiety. In taking out his frustrations on the nurse, the patient is not trying to be deliberately offensive, he is simply misattributing the source of his feelings and, therefore, misdirecting his response (which is manifested in anger toward the hospital nurse). It is extremely important for nurses to understand such responses so as not to take any such diatribes personally, and to remain calm and professional in dealing with such highly vulnerable patients.

*Being aware of Attribution Theory can assist in replacing judgmental attitudes with greater understanding, patience, and compassion.*

## CONCLUSION

A wise adage is to "believe nothing of what you hear and only half of what you see." While seemingly an amusing comment, this is in fact grounded in the psychological paradigm that, ultimately, there is no reality, only perception. How individuals perceive, interpret, and respond to stimuli in their environment often says a lot more about them than the situation in which they are involved. There are often more than two sides to every story and, therefore, nurses must be willing to reappraise, seek extra guidance, and accept that, in the face of further evidence, their beliefs may be wrong.

Becoming consciously aware of, and learning to overcome, common human errors of judgment will put nurses in a much stronger position to succeed in the challenging environment of modern medicine. Being conscious of their own attributions and their misattributions of others, in addition to theories about cause and effect, can impact on how resilient a nurse can be in the face of adversity and, in addition, how well a patient or client can approach their own self-care and recovery.

## LEARNING ACTIVITIES

This chapter explored the functional impact of different appraisals and reactive styles, which can sometimes lead to common human errors of judgment in highly stressful situations. The following three activities are designed to help you explore your own reactive style, the nature of physiological arousal, and the functional impact of reappraisals.

1. This self-test can help raise awareness of your own reactive style:

Raise your awareness about your explanatory style by rating, on a scale of 1 to 4, how much do you agree with the following statements? (1 = not at all; 4 = very much so)
- If I fail a test, I am certain it's my fault.
- Most people are inherently good.
- It's hard to really trust most people, because you never know what their real agenda is.
- I can easily overcome most of life's setbacks and obstacles.
- The world is becoming a more dangerous place.
- I feel confident about my future and the future of humankind in general.

If you agree more closely with the odd-numbered statements, your explanatory style tends to be more pessimistic; if you agree more closely with the even-numbered statements, your style is more optimistic. If your answers are mainly in the middle, your style is somewhere between the two on the continuum.

2. The following activity helps you reflect on the functional impact of different appraisals and their own reactive style:

In three or four sentences, describe a stressful situation that you have been in and how you reacted. Write a paragraph on how your explanatory style as assessed in this chapter is likely to have affected your attributions and appraisals. Can you articulate how your explanatory style might explain part of your reaction to this situation? In retrospect, what could you have done better to improve the functional outcome of this situation?

3. The final activity can help you understand the nature of physiological arousal and to consider how you might appraise challenging situations differently to avoid taking things personally and getting upset.

Consider and discuss these scenarios with your classmates:

- Imagine two people are pointing at you at a shopping center and laughing. You check your hair and make sure you haven't spilled anything on yourself but can find nothing wrong. What next? Do you still assume they are laughing at you? At this point, what other reappraisals of this situation can you generate? Perhaps, they were laughing at something behind you or in your vicinity. Perhaps, one was gesturing as part of telling a joke and not pointing at you at all. Even if they were laughing at you, perhaps, it was for reasons not as sinister as you think—maybe you have a picture on your T-shirt that reminds them of a situation they were in together that was hysterically funny. See how many reappraisals you can generate. Write down the different emotional responses and reactions each causes.
- An older adult patient makes a complaint against you of "mistreatment" during a recent attack of angina. He claims you were unnecessarily rough and demanding in ordering him to take his emergency medication and while taking his blood pressure. From the patient's point of view, what attributions and appraisals may have led to this complaint? How could you respond to this complaint in a functional manner?
- A doctor directs you to perform a procedure of which you have no knowledge or experience. Generate five different appraisals to explain why the doctor has requested you to do this. With reference to your list of appraisals, what are some functional ways to respond to this request?

## REFERENCES

Dutton, D. G., & Aron, A. P. (1974). Some evidence for heightened sexual attraction under conditions of high anxiety. *Journal of Personality and Social Psychology, 30*(4), 510–517. doi:10.1037/h0037031

Dykema, J., Bergbower, K., & Peterson, C. (1995). Pessimistic explanatory style, stress and illness. *Journal of Social and Clinical Psychology, 14*(4), 357–371. doi:10.1521/jscp.1995.14.4.357

Jackson, B., Sellers, R. M., & Peterson, C. (2002). Pessimistic explanatory style moderates the effect of stress on physical illness. *Personality and Individual Differences, 32*(3), 567–573. doi:10.1016/S0191-8869(01)00061-7

Keinan, G. (1987). Decision making under stress: Scanning of alternatives under controllable and uncontrollable conditions. *Journal of Personality and Social Psychology, 52*(3), 639–644. doi:10.1037/0022-3514.52.3.639

Lazarus, R. S. (1983). The costs and benefits of denial. In S. Bresznitz (Ed.), *The denial of stress* (pp. 1–32). New York, NY: Oxford University Press.

Martin-Krumm, C. P., Sarrazin, P. G., Peterson, C., & Famose, J.-P. (2003). Explanatory style and resilience after sports failure. *Personality and Individual Differences, 35*(7), 1685–1695. doi:10.1016/S0191-8869(02)00390-2

Peterson, C. (2000). The future of optimism. *American Psychologist, 55*(1), 45–55. doi:10.1037/0003-066X.55.1.44

Peterson, C., Seligman, M. E. P., & Vaillant, G. E. (1988). Pessimistic explanatory style is a risk factor for physical illness: A thirty-five year longitudinal study. *Journal of Personality and Social Psychology, 55*(1), 23–27. doi:10.1037/0022-3514.55.1.23

Pham, M. T. (2007). Emotion and rationality: A critical review and interpretation of empirical evidence. *Review of General Psychology, 11*(2), 155–178. doi:10.1037/1089-2680.11.2.155

Rule, B. G., & Nesdale, A. R. (1976). Emotional arousal and aggressive behaviour. *Psychological Bulletin, 83*(5), 851–863. doi:10.1037/0033-2909.83.5.851

Seo, M.-G., & Barrett, L. F. (2007). Being emotional during decision making: Good or bad? An empirical investigation. *Academy of Management Journal, 54*(4), 923–940. doi:10.5465/amj.2007.26279217

Taylor, S. E., & Brown, J. D. (1988). Illusion and well-being: A social psychological perspective on mental health. *Psychological Bulletin, 103*(2), 193–210. doi:10.1037/0033-2909.103.2.193

Tennen, H., & Affleck, G. (1987). The costs and benefits of optimistic explanations and dispositional optimism. *Journal of Personality, 55*(2), 377–393. doi:10.1111/j.1467-6494.1987.tb00443.x

White, G. L., Fishbein, S., & Rutstein, J. (1981). Passionate love and the misattribution of arousal. *Journal of Personality and Social Psychology, 41*(1), 56–62. doi:10.1037/0022-3514.41.1.56

Wild, J., Clark, E. M., Ehlers, A., & McManus, F. (2006). Perception of arousal in social anxiety: Effects of false feedback during a social interaction. *Journal of Behavior Therapy and Experimental Psychiatry, 39*(2), 102–116. doi:10.1016/j.jbtep.2006.11.003

# 7

# Building Resilience in Challenging Healthcare Situations

## Kim Foster and Andrew Estefan

### INTRODUCTION

A holistic or ecological view of health and well-being requires that nurses appreciate not only what may be affecting a person physically, but also psychologically, socially, environmentally, and politically. People with healthcare problems are social beings and are living with many strengths as well as vulnerabilities. In the contemporary world of nursing practice, nurses need to relate with their patients in a spirit of cooperation and collaborative partnership. This chapter draws upon two stories to explore resilient, collaborative actions, and practices nurses can use with patients who have complex health and social needs. Each story is discussed in respect to resilience and salutogenic theory (focusing on what supports health and well-being, rather than what causes illness and disease) and the application of resilient practices. The chapter begins with the story of a nurse working alongside the Maddison family, including Maya who has major depression and diabetes and is the mother of two children.

## THE MADDISON FAMILY'S STORY

Maya is 36 years old and is of Greek cultural heritage. She has experienced episodes of severe depression since her early 20s. She also has type 1 diabetes, which was diagnosed when she was 18. At that time, Maya, her parents, and the rest of her family were very distressed by her diagnosis, and Maya thought she would never have a normal life or have children. She now lives with Mike, her partner, and two children, Isabella (aged 8) and Alexander (aged 6). Mike and Maya have been together for 9 years, but lately have been having problems in their relationship due to Maya's ill health; they have been arguing a lot and Mike has been finding it difficult to cope. He has also been drinking more. He told Maya that he needs some time out and wants to move out from their home.

Maya has been attending the same general practice for several years for both herself and her children and has a good relationship with the nurses in the practice. A week ago, Maya was discharged from hospital after treatment for her latest episode of depression. She had been severely depressed and had psychotic symptoms including beliefs that her stomach was dead and hearing voices of her long-dead ancestors telling her to cut her stomach out. A week later, Maya still has a depressed mood, although her psychotic symptoms have reduced. She is taking antipsychotic and antidepressant medication and has come to the practice for review of her insulin dosage as her blood glucose levels have been very unstable for some weeks.

There is a mental health nurse working in primary healthcare who has worked with Maya over the past year and developed a good rapport with her. This nurse meets with her after she has had her blood glucose tested. She sees Maya is looking very down and asks how she is. Maya tells the nurse she has been discharged from a psychiatric unit again and starts to cry. She says she is worried it is all too much for Mike and the kids and that she is sick of being sick. The nurse listens quietly, letting her cry and talk about her concerns. She acknowledges her sadness, and also her courage in persevering with treatment for her depression and diabetes even though at times she feels like giving up. The nurse admires her commitment to Mike and her children even when she is unwell and tells her so. She also asks Maya what helps her when she is feeling down.

Together, Maya and the nurse discuss what would be most helpful for her in her current situation. They agree that it would be helpful for Maya to meet with the general practitioner (GP) that day to discuss her depression and medications. The nurse also agrees with Maya that another appointment needs to be made with the GP for Mike and Maya to discuss Mike's concerns about Maya's health and ways that he and Maya could be supported. The nurse also asks about the things Maya likes but has not been able to do since her recent illness. Maya tells the nurse that she would like to rejoin her basketball team, which meets weekly, as she has several friends in the team and feels better when she gets out of the house and exercises. Maya has kept a journal for many years, so the nurse also suggests she reflects each day on something she considers a strength of hers and writes it in her journal.

Two weeks later, the nurse sees Maya again when she comes for a follow-up of her blood glucose levels. She notes that Maya's mood had improved but she still lacks energy. Maya tells the nurse that she and Mike had met with the GP and talked about Maya's health and Mike's concerns. Mike indicated he still wanted a break and would be moving out for a while, but also that he remained committed to Maya and the children and would continue to see them regularly. Maya was very upset about this but felt it had been good to talk about it with someone else and she and Mike had agreed to go to relationship counseling while they were separated. Maya had also gone to one of her basketball team practice sessions and had enjoyed seeing her friends.

The nurse listened carefully to Maya and acknowledged her follow-through of the strategies they had discussed and encouraged her to continue with these. The nurse also asked if there was any support Maya needed during that time. Maya told the nurse that she would like to continue seeing her when she came in for her diabetes management. She was also concerned about the effect of her and Mike's separation and her latest episode of depression on Isabella and Alexander. In response, the nurse gave Maya some contact information for a local family support service, and a "flip" book with information for parents with mental health problems on one side, and key messages for their school-aged children on the other side that parents and children can discuss together. She also suggested that Maya bring the children in with her next time and they could all have a chat together about any questions or concerns they might have about their dad not being at home, and their mom being unwell.

## COMPLEX HEALTH PROBLEMS AND RESILIENCE

The Maddison family's story illustrates the type of complex health problems that many families experience and shows the opportunity for nurses to work with individuals and families in the prevention of physical and mental health conditions, treatment adherence, lifestyle changes, social support, and sustaining the connections those individuals and families have within the community. While Maya might be the patient, the nursing focus is also on the family unit, particularly the children. This is important because, not only do individuals within a family have their own health vulnerabilities and strengths, the family system itself is impacted. From a biological perspective, Maya has a long-term physical condition—type 1 diabetes—that is associated with shortened life expectancy and health complications in many body systems. From a psychological perspective, Maya has a severe and recurring mental illness. From a social and family perspective, Maya has current relationship problems and is a parent to two young children. In all these domains, Maya's health and well-being can be influenced for better or worse by her environment—including her relationships and social supports, the meeting of basic needs including housing and food, and access to resources including healthcare, education, and work. That is, complex health conditions are influenced by what are known as the social determinants of health—the conditions within which people are born, live, develop, and work (World Health Organization [WHO], 2018). Social determinants include poverty, conflict, stigma, and unstable living conditions. These determinants are shaped by the distribution of power, wealth, and resources in societies (WHO, 2018), and are responsible for health inequities, which can exacerbate mental and physical health challenges, in this case not only for Maya but for her entire family.

Along with Maya's ongoing mental health problem, the children's mental health is paramount. Children can be at risk of developing major mental disorders if they experience disruptions to parental care and support during their early years (Van der Kolk, 2017). Children whose parents have a mental illness are at risk of developing their own mental health problems due to various factors. These include the psychosocial impacts of mental illness on parents and the family (such as poverty and lack of housing), as well as the potential effects of parents' mental illness on their parenting and relationship with their children (such as psychosis or abusive behaviors), and the child's genetic vulnerability to mental illness and personal characteristics (such as temperament type, intelligence, physical illness, or disabilities; Foster, O'Brien, & Korhonen, 2012). The partners of people with co-associated physical and mental illness, such as Mike, are also impacted by their caring roles and are known to experience higher physical and emotional strain than other partners (Hastrup, Van den Berg, & Gyrd-Hansen, 2011) and may be vulnerable to developing their own mental health and substance use problems. Clearly, everyone in Maya's family is in need of support.

Complex health conditions are those where multiple morbidities combine—in Maya's case these involve the physical health challenges of diabetes control and her mental health challenges and vulnerabilities, as well as the mental health risks to her children. She also has issues of social need such as of parenting support, and relationship counseling (Kuluski, Ho, Hans, & Nelson, 2017). Other examples of health conditions that can be considered complex include arthritis, respiratory disease, cardiac disease, chronic kidney disease, and cancer. These conditions are often co-associated with other conditions, particularly depression, and this can lead to physical and/or psychological disability and social disadvantage (New South Wales [NSW] Government, Family & Community Services, 2014). Maya's story shows how complex health conditions are often persistent and need ongoing intervention to prevent problems before they occur, or to identify and resolve problems before they develop further. Her story also shows how complex health conditions can have long-lasting and far-reaching consequences for those they affect. The need for complex healthcare is based on two key aspects of complex health conditions: their impact and their severity (NSW Government, Family & Community Services, 2014).

*The need for complex healthcare is based on two key aspects of complex health conditions: their impact and their severity.*

Nurses who practice in a variety of healthcare contexts are well positioned to exert positive influence on the impact and severity of patients' complex health problems and, in the process, to help strengthen patients' resilience. All nurses can cultivate relational practices (i.e., nursing practice that is based on the connection or relationship built with patients) built around their knowledge of the patient, an understanding of the contextual and relational complexities that intersect the patient's experiences of their health, and working positively and adaptively toward sustainable and meaningful health promotion. As Edward (2013) notes, nurses can help patients resist the stress of complex health conditions through using existing nursing skills such as early intervention. This includes making an assessment of a person's social supports and coping strategies, assisting to support a positive family climate, encouraging peer involvement (e.g., interacting with friends), and making referrals to community services such as mothers' or church groups.

Nurses in primary healthcare (i.e., the first layer of healthcare services such as in general practices and private practices) particularly have the potential to work with patients to help them make positive adaptations to their lifestyle and personal health practices (Keleher et al., 2007). Nurses in specializations like mental health and psychiatric nursing can assist patients to manage the competing demands that affect the balance of their mental and physical health (Blakeman & Ford, 2012; Warelow & Edward, 2007). All these nurses can cooperate and work together within, and across, services by sharing their expertise in order to provide comprehensive care for their patients and families. In the Maddison family's story, for example, the mental health nurse brings mental and psychosocial health expertise and strategies. This is complemented by the practice nurse's expertise in general nursing care, which can, in turn, be further complemented by liaising with a diabetes nurse who has specialist knowledge in the physiology, assessment, and management of type 1 diabetes.

Individuals with co-associated illnesses, as well as their children and partners, can be supported to build their individual and family resilience through individual, family, and social strategies and resources, and nurses play a key role in facilitating this resilience building. The value of employing mental health nurses to work alongside practice nurses and doctors in general practice settings is clear within the Maddison family's story. These nurses are trained in being alert to mental health issues across the life span. In primary health, their role involves working with patients who have complex physical and mental health conditions. Nurses, therefore, require finely tuned bio-psycho-social-spiritual skills. They plan patient care, review patients' mental state, monitor their medication, and link patients with other service providers and services (Meehan & Robertson, 2013). In the Maddison family's story, the mental health nurse used a range of interpersonal strategies to support Maya including empathic listening, reflection of feelings, reflection of content of talk, and validation. The conversations the nurse had with Maya were also solution-focused—the nurse took a proactive approach to Maya's health and well-being that emphasized and built upon Maya's strengths (e.g., her perseverance, courage in dealing with her health challenges, her commitment to her children and partner), and resources (e.g., her family support, the GP and practice nurses, her basketball team and friends), and recognized that her resilience was as important as her vulnerabilities (McAllister, 2010).

*A solution-focused nursing approach is consistent with a social–ecological view of resilience as it focuses not only on the individual, but on their sociocultural world (McAllister, 2010).*

There is growing evidence that resilience is an important factor in the process and outcomes of complex health problems. A solution-focused nursing approach is consistent with a socioecological view of resilience as it focuses not only on the individual, but on their sociocultural world (McAllister, 2010). Systematic review findings indicate that higher resilience is associated with fewer mental health problems and better quality of life for people with chronic health conditions. Conversely, lower resilience is associated with poorer mental health, greater illness progression, and difficulty controlling blood glucose levels (Cal, de Sa, Glustak, & Santiago, 2015). For people like Maya with diabetes, resilience (defined in this particular study as possessing the positive psychosocial resources of self-efficacy, optimism, self-mastery, and self-esteem) has been found to buffer the effects of rising psychological distress on self-care behaviors and blood glucose control (Yi, Vitaliano, Smith, Yi, & Weinger, 2008). Wister et al. (2016) argue that a whole-of-life approach to resilience is needed for multimorbid conditions, as these complex conditions can have cumulative effects over time. A whole-of-life approach links past health and illness experiences with the person's present personal and environmental context.

Taking a social ecological perspective on resilience is relevant to understanding complex health conditions, because, as illustrated by the example of the Maddison family, these conditions challenge people in every aspect of their life. In this way of thinking, resilience becomes less about a person's individual characteristics and more about the interactive processes that occur between that person and the environment or ecology. This involves nurses and other caregivers being able to find resources that help sustain their well-being, and the ability of their environment—including family, healthcare professionals and services, workplaces, and other community organizations—to provide them (Ungar, 2008, 2011). With complex health conditions, resilient processes are those that help people recover and restore their well-being through using their personal resources (e.g., self-efficacy, problem solving, optimism), in conjunction with accessing practical, financial, emotional, social, and healthcare support from the people and services around them (Masten & Obradovic, 2006). Together, this mutual interaction can result in resilient outcomes for individuals and families, such as well-being and recovery. This means that this perspective on resilience in complex health conditions is not focused on the individual alone but includes a range of other people and resources that are needed to help people adapt in challenging circumstances. Figure 7.1 shows how each of these types of resources can interact.

## RESILIENCE IN ACTION

*Resilient practice is more than practical action; resilient practices are those where nurses also draw on their mental, emotional, and practical knowledge and skills to respond effectively to others in challenging healthcare situations (Foster, Cuzzillo, & Furness, 2018).*

Nurses are often focused on practical actions that can help patients and their families deal with the healthcare challenges they face.

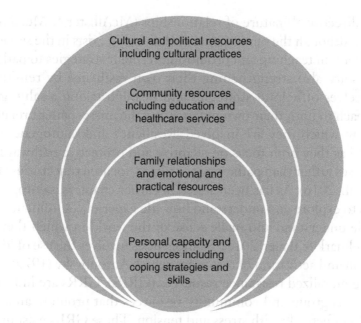

**Figure 7.1** Socioecological resilience.

Resilient practice is more than practical action, however; resilient practices are those where nurses also draw on their mental, emotional, and practical knowledge and skills to respond effectively to others in challenging healthcare situations (Foster et al., 2018). Being able to manage powerful negative emotions such as anger or anxiety, being able to be empathetic toward others even when their behavior is challenging, and acknowledging and managing negative thoughts in stressful situations, are examples of resilient practices nurses have used to manage difficult interactions with clients and colleagues (Foster et al., 2018). These are skills that can be learned and, therefore, also taught to others including patients, through role modeling and direct skills teaching. As in the Maddison family's story, mental health nurses, for instance, focus particularly on people's subjective mental and emotional experiences, and use their own mental and emotional skills to understand these experiences and to help the person with practical strategies to prevent or manage distress.

From an ecological perspective, resilience can be developed in nurses as well as their patients through understanding the mutual (or bidirectional) nature of relationships (McAllister & McKinnon, 2008). Although the nurse–patient relationship exists in the service of the client, in teaching and promoting resilient strategies to patients, nurses are also strengthening their own resilience by reminding themselves of helpful strategies and through taking a salutogenic approach to both their own practice and the nurse–patient relationships in which they are involved. Resilience and salutogenesis are related as they both focus on adaptive and protective pathways and processes rather than pathogenic or illness-focused trajectories (Wister et al., 2016). As has been stated in earlier chapters, salutogenesis helps to explore and understand how life experiences influence how people understand and make sense of the world in which they live (Mittelmark & Bauer, 2017). Salutogenesis involves the use of identification and activation of resources, which Antonovsky (1979) refers to as generalized resistance resources (GRRs). GRRs are individual as well as group and community resources that promote an ability to deal effectively with stress and tension. These GRRs exist in tension with generalized resistance deficits, meaning that a person can be understood to be on a continuum of adaptive coping and deficit coping (Idan, Eriksson, & Al-Yagon, 2017). At an individual level, attachments, childhood experiences, family supports, social support, and genetics are GRRs that contribute to varying levels of adaptation and coping. Family influences include family atmosphere, geographical distribution of family, parenting style, and family socioeconomic status. Social GRRs are those that arise through engagement with schools, workplaces, social supports, and friendship groups.

The salutogenic model proposes a relationship between GRRs and another phenomenon, or attribute, called "sense of coherence" (Antonovsky, 1987). A person's sense of coherence describes a feeling of comfortable fit with events occurring in that person's world and their meaning. This sense arises through three principal mechanisms: being able to understand what is happening; believing that whatever is happening is something that can be dealt with; and the ability to find meaning in what is happening and integrate it into one's overall stream of experience. Antonovsky (1979) termed these mechanisms comprehensibility, manageability, and meaningfulness. Alongside the GRRs, these mechanisms work to moderate the sense of whether or not a person is coping with, and adapting to, challenges or change.

Together, these salutogenic processes can help people maintain their health and to thrive in challenging circumstances (Stock, 2017). The processes that apply for people in challenging health circumstances may be both similar, and different, to those that apply to nurses working with patients. Regardless of differing GRRs and different influences on sense of coherence, the nurse–patient encounter is a rich context in which to explore a resilience-informed relationship that has beneficial and positive outcomes for patients and nurses. Having positive relationships with and support from others, sustaining passion for what you do, and personal characteristics including sense of humor and confidence are examples of salutogenesis in action (Stock, 2017).

> *Having positive relationships with and support from others, sustaining passion for what you do, and personal characteristics including sense of humor and confidence are examples of salutogenesis in action (Stock, 2017).*

## BUILDING RESILIENCE IN COMPLEX SITUATIONS

The discussion so far has emphasized that effective coping is a key feature of resilient responses to stress and adversity. In healthcare, these coping strategies can be reinforced by all members in a multidisciplinary team who can share the problems and solutions across their specialty areas. In Table 7.1, we draw upon the idea of individual, family, and social GRRs to show some differences between healthy and unhealthy coping strategies that have been identified through research. These are relevant to the Maddison family's story as well as Jaden's story that follows.

The examples of coping strategies used by Maya and Mike in the Maddison family's story indicate complexity and require sensitive, empathetic considerations. For some patients, rather than being healthy or making adaptive strategies, talking with family members or engaging in some types of exercise or relaxation can be risky and diminish the client's sense of coherence or access to resources and, therefore, the client's ability to cope. People can expand their repertoire of effective ways to cope with stress and health challenges through being taught effective strategies, and through making healthy

**Table 7.1** Healthy and Unhealthy Coping Strategies

| Adaptive (Healthy) Coping Strategies | Maladaptive (Unhealthy) Coping Strategies |
|---|---|
| Talking with friends and family | Abusing alcohol and/or drugs |
| Exercising regularly | Overeating or undereating |
| Talking with a counselor | Gambling |
| Religious or spiritual practices | Smoking |
| Relaxation and/or meditation | Isolating from others |
| Seeing the humor in situations | Ongoing conflict between parents |
| Letting others help | Stealing |
| Taking strength from past experiences | Over- or under-sleeping |
| Having hope for the future | |

Source: Adapted from West, C., Stewart, L., Foster, K., & Usher, K. (2012). The meaning of resilience to persons living with chronic pain: An interpretive qualitative inquiry. Journal of Clinical Nursing, 21(9–10), 1284–1292. doi:10.1111/j.1365-2702.2011.04005.x

resources more available to them (Holton, Barry, & Chaney, 2016), but in order to help patients accomplish this, nurses need to gain important insights into patients' circumstances. Insights into a family's holistic life circumstances contribute to resilient practice by sustaining a socioecological perspective. In this way, it is possible for nurses to consider broader factors that influence the impact and severity of complex health conditions. These important insights contribute to a broader plan of care in which the nurse–patient relationship becomes the context and grounding for exploration of experiences and the movement toward resilient outcomes.

*Insights into a family's holistic life circumstances contribute to resilient practice by sustaining a socioecological perspective.*

Many nurses have been socialized into a practice that is deficit-based (Doyle et al., 2018), and nursing practice continues to be understood as an assistive practice to the discipline of medicine, which is oriented on pathology and medical treatments to solve health problems (McAllister, Moyle, & Iselin, 2006). For those nurses who wish to extend their practice toward also being oriented to a health-adaptation, growth, and strength-based practice, solution-focused approaches can be challenging to do because they are not a natural first course of action (Lind & Smith, 2008). Nurses are taught to focus on problems, and the systems in which nurses work often emphasize disease- or illness-focused approaches to care. As well, working in ways that influence and develop resilience requires a shift in the nurse–patient relationship that can reduce nurses' sense of mastery or control over their practice. This is because the development of resilient practice necessitates the activation of different skills or qualities of practice from a deficit-based approach. In the deficit-based approach, clinicians are the expert and dispense prescriptive interventions, drawn mainly from evidence-based techniques. They tend to be impartial, distant, and objective. But in a resilience-based collaborative approach, clinicians—including nurses—use deeper engagement, imagination, collaboration, and therapeutic risk-taking. In the latter approach, the nurse–patient relationship is being developed in the midst of a different kind of agenda: one that develops as a way to hold the patient up, to identify motivators, inspire endurance, and build capacity, rather than "fix" the patient's problems.

The following case study, that we have entitled Jaden's story, illustrates both this complexity and possibility for nursing. Jaden is a university student who initially presents with physical health symptoms that unfold into a more complex presentation. His story illustrates the complexities of health problems and also the potential for alternate explanations for patients' presenting symptoms.

## JADEN'S STORY

Jaden is a 25-year-old man who is in his first year of studying law to gain his Juris Doctor degree. Like his classmates, this is Jaden's second degree, his first being a dual degree in history and international relations. He graduated magna cum laude from his first degree and was accepted into law that same year. Since starting his law degree, Jaden has been living away from his hometown for the first time.

The nurse first met Jaden 3 weeks into the beginning of the academic year, when he came to the university health clinic, where the nurse works as a primary health nurse. Jaden came to the university health clinic to, he said, rather ambiguously, get "checked out." He was dressed casually but took care in his appearance. He was clean shaven, wore jeans, a hoodie, and a baseball cap indicating he supported the university's football team. At the first meeting, the nurse did a comprehensive intake assessment, including a head-to-toe assessment, blood glucose test, and urinalysis. Jaden's vital signs were normal. His temperature was 98.8°F (37.1°C), his blood pressure was 128/77 mmHg, his heart rate was a regular 76 beats per minute, and he was breathing normally. The assessment suggested he was neurologically stable and, when asked, he reported that he had had no recent falls or head injury. The blood glucose test result was 5.9 mmol/L (postprandial) and the urinalysis showed only slightly elevated specific gravity. Talking more with Jaden, the nurse learned that he was living in the university residence, along a corridor that housed a mixture of undergraduate students, most of whom were studying in engineering and humanities programs. When asked specifically, he advised that he had made friends with, as he said, "a couple of people" in his law program, but otherwise most of his social life remained back in his hometown. Jaden described his relationships with his parents and sister as "loving" but "strained at times."

Jaden said that over the previous few days he had been feeling nauseous, and despite not vomiting, the nausea remained persistent. He also reported that he had been experiencing headaches for the last 4 to 5 weeks and felt they were getting worse. When asked about the location and type of pain, Jaden said they were "just headaches" but that he had been needing to take over-the-counter painkillers (acetaminophen/paracetamol or ibuprofen) at least once a day for them. The nurse referred Jaden to the clinic's nurse practitioner (NP) who performed a comprehensive assessment, including: abdominal palpation of liver, spleen, and rebound tenderness; signs of benign paroxysmal vertigo; evidence of concussion; examination of Jaden's ears for infection; and assessment for gastroesophageal reflux disease. The NP determined these were unlikely causes of the nausea and headaches: Jaden had no fever; he was not in pain or guarding his abdomen; his liver was normal size; and his spleen was nonpalpable. Jaden reported no history of diarrhea or abdominal cramping and the NP found no other symptoms of food poisoning. Although Jaden did not describe his headaches as severe, the NP asked him if he had experienced any prodromal, aural, or postdromal symptoms of migraine. Jaden responded that he thought he had seen a "weird shape" in front of his eyes "once or twice" before.

Jaden told the NP that he had been preoccupied with getting on top of his coursework and so had not been taking much care with what he had been eating and drinking. He had also been attempting to socialize at the university and had become intoxicated on several nights over the course of the first weeks of semester. One of these incidents he did not remember very well. The NP noted in the chart that Jaden presented with tension headache and possible migraine symptoms. The NP discussed with Jaden ways to manage his headaches and nausea as well as how to embed effective self-care, including adequate hydration in his university routine. The NP requested a blood test for liver function and fasting glucose, and wrote a referral to the student support service so that Jaden could obtain access to the academic and personal resources that could help him manage better in the early weeks and months of his law degree.

Two weeks later, Jaden made another appointment with the university health service. He spoke briefly with the intake receptionist who then asked the nurse to urgently assess Jaden. The receptionist said Jaden was vague about his symptoms, but that Jaden was worried it could be serious. When the nurse assessed Jaden, he was complaining of headache, nausea, and more generalized pain. The nurse found him to be less talkative than on his first attendance; he shared less information about his studies and his social life. Jaden told the nurse that he had spoken to his sister yesterday and she had told him that she missed having him at home and she was worried about him. He spoke at some length about his growing concern that his headaches and nausea had not diminished, and that he felt "achey," like he might be getting the flu. The nurse's assessment showed he was afebrile but he did have a slightly elevated heart rate (94 bpm) and his blood pressure was high, too (150/88). There were no other obvious signs of illness or injury and Jaden was cooperative, although quiet, throughout the assessment. The nurse reviewed Jaden's chart and noted that the results of the blood tests, requested by the NP, are all normal. The NP examined him within the hour and found no other obvious cause for his symptoms.

As he left the office, the NP noticed Jaden's facial expression and decided to go up and talk to him again. After some preliminary small talk about how the last couple of weeks have been for him, Jaden told the nurse that he had been drunk most nights in his room in the residence and wondered aloud whether this was why he felt unwell. The nurse agreed with him that there could be a connection and invited him to sit down. The nurse asked him if he felt able to say more. Over the course of another 40 minutes, Jaden talked about being on the cusp of "tapping out" (voluntarily withdrawing from his course), and that he was on a trajectory toward failing. He said that he had found it harder to make friends and connections at university than he thought he would. He described moments of feeling "brave and invincible" and during these times he would go out with the intent of being sociable, but that usually came to a "screeching halt" with the realization that he just did not fit in. In contrast to these moments of feeling brave, Jaden experienced other times when he felt "filled with dread" at the thought of having to learn his course work, participate in class discussion, and produce assignment work. He went on to say that he found himself crying "more than I ever have in my life" and that drinking dampened down the sadness and worry that he was not doing well. Jaden had, he said, spent many nights like this in his room. He described a usual pattern of finishing his classes for the day and dreading the evening, then walking to the market to buy either a bottle of vodka or rum, and returning to his room to drink it, watch television and eventually fall asleep. Jaden criticized himself for "binge watching" old episodes of a science fiction series he used to like when he was a teenager; with an ironic laugh he said, "It's like they are my only friends these days."

The night before this discussion, he admitted he did not have enough money to buy anything to drink and he stole a bottle of rum from the store. It was the first time he had stolen anything, and he said he realized the significance of it. Although he was not caught, the impulsiveness of the decision to steal the rum frightened him. The nurse asked Jaden if anyone else was aware of what is happening with him. He told the nurse that, on several occasions, he had shared his loneliness and social struggles with his sister. She called him regularly and, although Jaden said he "loves that she is concerned," he also found her concern, and her questions, intrusive. The day before, Jaden's parents had called because his sister had told them how he was doing. His parents suggested that they travel down and stay in town to help him "sort himself out." Jaden does not want them to come because he thinks if they do he will lose control over what happens next.

## GOING BEYOND PRESENTING PROBLEMS

Practicing nursing with complex conditions from a socioecological resilience perspective means venturing out, alongside patients, past the problems they present with and into conversations about how these individuals are making meaning of their health and illness experiences. The nurse in Jaden's story noticed that he was unsettled, perhaps unhappy, when he left the NP's office. Taking the time to speak with Jaden created an opportunity for him to take a risk and disclose more about his circumstances. Jaden's presenting problems of headache and nausea needed to be assessed and treated where appropriate but allowing him to speak about what else was happening for him began to allow for other insights and experiences to inform the therapeutic relationship.

Jaden's headache and nausea were real experiences for him, but he also needed a different kind of care. Attending only to his presenting medical problems would mean that the possibility for this kind of care would be foreclosed. Jaden knew that he was struggling in some aspects of university life, and recognized that he was beginning to form negative patterns and habits that were also unhelpful in terms of being successful at university. Although he had been trying different strategies to manage and cope, Jaden was beginning to feel like he was running out of options.

Jaden's story serves as a reminder that it is easy to take an individualistic view of resilience, but his circumstances are more complex and necessitate a more expansive lens. Jaden is both vulnerable and coping. His vulnerabilities are social/relational and individual. Jaden is aware that being away from home is harder than he expected. He also recognizes that he has not yet developed workable strategies for managing his coursework. He has begun to retreat, to drink alcohol, and he has not, until his visit to the clinic, shared his experiences with anyone other than his sister. Although his family is a source of coping, Jaden worries that they will take control of his situation. His story can be read as a conventional one of maladjustment, ineffective coping, anxiety, and substance use. Jaden's experience is, however, also a rich source of information about possibilities and capacities for resilience, and resilient practice.

Although Jaden tells his story as one in which many things are going wrong, there are also several aspects of his experience that reveal his capacities and resilience. For example, he has a history and track record of academic success. Graduating magna cum laude means Jaden was in the top 10% of his graduating class in his previous dual degree. Close attention to Jaden's story reveals that his sense of failing to be a successful student independent of his previous hometown context was greater than the risk of failing coursework. Although he had expressed anxiety about his coursework, this was not the central focus for Jaden.

There are also glimpses of adventurousness in Jaden's story. He has shown that he can take helpful, as well as harmful, risks. On the one hand, he has moved away from familiar places and people, to venture into a graduate-entry law degree. He has taken steps to socialize but this has not been an entirely satisfying or successful experience for him. He has described moments of enthusiasm and interest in making connections, tempered with times where he has retreated from these efforts. Using a conventional, problem orientation, the retreat from challenging circumstances can be thought of as a failure to adapt (Boyd & Mackey, 2000). Such a view can, however, be unhelpful because it individualizes social issues, making them the problems of the people involved. Indeed, when people run away from their problems, conventional wisdom advises that those problems often go with them because they have not been solved. A resilience perspective informed by a socioecological view makes it possible to understand this dynamic differently. Taking oneself to a different context, away from particular tension and complexity, can be a resilience factor. Recognizing that different places, even dormitory bedrooms, offer different wisdom and possibilities for self means that mobility, movement, and even retreat are adaptive options that can be explored in nurse–patient relationships (Estefan & Roughley, 2013). Jaden's retreat from challenging circumstances was not absolute. His willingness to talk to his family, even in the context of that relationship sometimes being strained, suggests that he recognized some of the resources that help him sort through some of his problems. He also sought care from the university health clinic, even though he first presented with what seemed to be physical health problems. Amid some of the difficult experiences he has had, Jaden showed he recognized some of the helpful people in his social world and that he can and will reach out.

Jaden's original presentation to the university clinic for headaches and flu-like symptoms might easily be read as him being unwilling or unable to talk about or explain what was happening for him. On the other hand, it shows him taking advantage of a resource. Perhaps presenting to the clinic with his physical symptoms helped Jaden determine whether it felt safe to disclose more information. When he decided to talk more openly about his experiences, he offered a candid account of what has been happening for him. He showed that he had the capacity to look inward in a self-facing way, and outward toward his social setting and relationships. Jaden showed courage in describing to the nurse how he was navigating a difficult path. This means that there exists an opportunity for helpful resilient practice to facilitate and strengthen this.

## RESILIENT PRACTICE FOR HEALTH AND WELL-BEING

In order to facilitate the development of resilience, a shift in focus is necessary. Although it might be tempting to think of Jaden's story as one of imminent failure at university, Jaden shows many signs of being able to succeed. Interventions that aim to prevent failure may proceed from a deficit perspective and, as such, not be able to recognize or capitalize on a person's strengths. Resilient practice can help patients sustain resilience-building when the broader institutional context might view them as in deficit and enact interventions accordingly, and thus nurses who practice in institutional contexts like universities need to be aware of the relationship patients have with their respective institutional contexts. Without intervention, over time, Jaden may have been identified by the university as being "at risk" of failing. That is to say, he may have shown diminished attendance, reduced participation, and poor grades. Intervention on the part of the university would focus on managing risk; Jaden would become the object of the university's interventions to help him succeed.

Viewed from a different perspective however, Jaden was not academically or even socially incapable, he can be seen to be—instead—out of place and not yet been able to feel a sense of fit with his new living, learning, and social environment. Much like many others in demanding professional university programs, Jaden had little room to explore who he was and who he was becoming (Estefan, Caine, & Clandinin, 2016), but what he was becoming was happening in a context that did not support it. It is here that the helpfulness of attending to sense of coherence (Antonovsky, 1987) becomes more obvious. By attending to the comprehensibility dimension of a personal sense of coherence, nurses can work with a person to help them make sense of the relationships between who they are and are becoming and the experiences they have. In this way, nurses can help patients to understand what is happening to, and around, them. As well, nurses can perform helpful work to strengthen patients' sense of how they can manage. Jaden, for instance, relied on familiar resources—his sister, his studiousness, his inclination to be sociable, and his capacity to identify helpful resources—that both affirmed and challenged who he was. Resilience-based therapeutic work in a nurse–patient relationship can help patients to think about, imagine, and experiment with new resources and increase capacity for coping. Importantly, this therapeutic work can support and extend understanding of self, capability, and capacity in the context of a person's relationship with broader social contexts that are variously constraining and facilitative. In this way, the nurse–patient relationship can become a context for the exploration of Antonovsky's (1987) third component of sense of coherence, meaningfulness.

## CONCLUSION

There exists for nurses an opportunity to make meaningful, therapeutic connections with patients that extend beyond the clinical encounter. Adopting a socioecological resilience perspective has two important implications for practice. First, it means that nurses must understand therapeutic relationships with patients as part of the patient's broader social context. Second, nurses need to think about each nurse–patient relationship as part of the broader social endeavor of nursing practice. In this way, nursing practice becomes both sustaining and a source of resilience for nurses because each nurse–patient relationship has something to contribute to nurses' understanding of how to cultivate their own meaningful individual practice (and practice identity) alongside building a community of nurses who, together, also participate in the social endeavor of nursing.

In this chapter, a social ecological resilience approach has framed the exploration of how nurses can work cooperatively with patients with complex health problems using resilient and salutogenic practices. An ecological view of health and well-being requires a holistic understanding of physical, psychological, social, environmental, and political resources that patients and nurses can access to build resilience in challenging healthcare situations. Working in partnership, patients and nurses are able to identify strengths as well as vulnerabilities and collaborate together to build and sustain patients' health and well-being in the face of complex and enduring health problems.

## LEARNING ACTIVITIES

1. From a social ecological perspective, discuss the personal (e.g., cognitive and emotional and coping strategies), social (e.g., family and friends), and environmental (including healthcare professionals and services, workplaces, and other community organizations) resources that could be accessed to support Maya, Mike, Isabella, and Alexander to achieve resilient outcomes in the challenging period of Maya's illness and recovery described in this chapter. What might a resilient outcome look like for Maya, Mike, Isabella, and Alexander?

2. What are some other GRRs (Antonovsky, 1979) that you might explore with Jaden, as you assess and develop a plan of care with him? In particular, what are some of the opportunities and constraints of understanding family as a GRR for Jaden?

3. **Creative Thinking Exercise**
   This exercise is in two parts. Part one: Either individually or with others ask yourself, "What is my/our immediate impression about Jaden's presentation and what is my/our attention drawn to first?" Then think about the professional knowledge, social messages, stories, and influences that shape your impression of Jaden. Part two: Now turn your attention to where you might see evidence of resilience in Jaden's story. Ask yourself some critical questions about why some of Jaden's resilience factors are easier to notice than others. Think about the relationship between how you think about resilience and the broader educational, social, perspectives you identified above.

4. **Education Activity**

   Identify a complex health problem (e.g., diabetes, paraplegia, and long-term mental illness) and consider the physical, psychological, and social adversities that are known to occur with this problem. Consider also how it may be possible to achieve a resilient outcome when the problem is ongoing. What factors and resources are needed to achieve a resilient outcome for the person? What would a resilient outcome look like for the person? How would the person and the nurse know they had achieved a resilient outcome? What do nurses need to know and do to help achieve a resilient outcome for a person with this problem?

5. **The next activity has three stages:**

   - Identify with learners some of the challenges that nurses can experience in composing their own resilient practice. For example, you might choose to explore practice in the context of institutional constraints, policy, horizontal violence, and workloads. You might also encourage learners to explore complex practice contexts.

   - Ask learners to think about and write down possibilities or opportunities for resilient practice in relation to the identified issues or practice contexts.

   - Invite learners to add to their list by thinking about how teams of nurses (or teams of nurses and other health professionals) can build *and sustain* resilient practices.

## REFERENCES

Antonovsky, A. (1979). *Health, stress, and coping*. San Francisco, CA: Jossey-Bass.

Antonovsky, A. (1987). *Unraveling the mystery of health*. San Francisco, CA: Jossey-Bass.

Blakeman, P., & Ford, L. (2012). Working in the real world: Review of sociological concepts of health and well-being and their relation to modern mental health nursing. *Journal of Psychiatric and Mental Health Nursing, 19*, 482–491. doi:10.1111/j.1365-2850.2011.01818.x

Boyd, M. R., & Mackey, M. C. (2000). Running away to nowhere: Rural women's experiences of becoming alcohol dependent. *Archives of Psychiatric Nursing, 14*(3), 142–149. doi:10.1053/py.2000.6385

Cal, S. F., de Sa, L., Glustak, M. E., Santiago, M. B. (2015). Resilience in chronic diseases: A systematic review. *Cogent Psychology, 2*, 1024928. doi:10.1080/23311908.2015.1024928

Doyle, L., Ellila, H., Jormfeldt, H., Lahti, M., Higgins, A., Keogh, B., . . . Kilkku, N. (2018). Preparing master-level mental health nurses to work within a wellness paradigm: Findings from the eMenthe project. *International Journal of Mental Health Nursing, 27*, 823–832. doi:10.1111/inm.12370

Edward, K.-L. (2013). Chronic illness and wellbeing: Using nursing practice to foster resilience as resistance. *British Journal of Nursing, 22*(13), 741–746. doi:10.12968/bjon.2013.22.13.741

Estefan, A., Caine, V., & Clandinin, D. J. (2016). At the intersections of narrative inquiry and professional education. *Narrative Works: Issues, Investigations, and Interventions, 6*(1), 15–37. Retrieved from https://journals.lib.unb.ca/index .php/NW/article/view/25444/29478

Estefan, A., & Roughley, R. A. (2013). Composing self on narrative landscapes of sexual difference: A story of wisdom and resilience. *Canadian Journal of Counselling and Psychotherapy, 47*(1), 29–48. Retrieved from https://cjc-rcc .ucalgary.ca/article/view/60125

Foster, K., Cuzzillo, C., & Furness, T. (2018). Strengthening mental health nurses' resilience through a workplace resilience program: A qualitative inquiry. *Journal of Psychiatric and Mental Health Nursing, 25*, 338–348. doi:10.1111/jpm.12467

Foster, K., O'Brien, L. & Korhonen, T. (2012). Developing resilient children and families where parents have mental illness: A family-focused approach. *International Journal of Mental Health Nursing, 21*(1), 3–11. doi:10.1111/j.1447-0349.2011.00754.x

Hastrup, L. H., Van den Berg, B., & Gyrd-Hansen, D. (2011). Do informal caregivers in mental illness feel more burdened? A comparative study of mental versus somatic illnesses. *Scandinavian Journal of Public Health, 39*, 598–607. doi:10.1177/1403494811414247

Holton, M. K., Barry, A. E., & Chaney, J. D. (2016). Employee stress management: An examination of adaptive and maladaptive coping strategies on employee health. *Work, 53*, 299–305. doi:10.3233/WOR-152145

Idan, O., Eriksson, M., & Al-Yagon, M. (2017). The salutogenic model: The role of generalized resistance resources. In M. B. Mittlemark, S. Sagy, M. Eriksson, G. F. Bauer, J. M. Pelikan, B. Lindstrom, & G. A. Espnes (Eds.), *The handbook of salutogenesis* (pp. 57–70). New York, NY: Springer.

Keleher, H., Parker, R., Abdulwadud, O., Francis, K., Segal, L., & Dalziel, K. (2007). *Review of primary and community care nursing.* Clayton, Victoria, Australia: Department of Health Science, Monash University.

Kuluski, K., Ho, J. W., Hans, P. K., & Nelson, M. L. A. (2017). Community care for people with complex care needs: Bridging the gap between health and social care. *International Journal of Integrated Care, 17*(4), 1–11. doi:10.5334/ ijic.2944

Lind, C., & Smith, D. (2008). Analyzing the state of community health nursing: Advancing from deficit to strengths-based practice using appreciative inquiry. *Advances in Nursing Science, 31*(1), 28–41. doi:10.1097/01.ANS.0000311527 .35446.4c

Masten, A., & Obradovic, J. (2006). Competence and resilience in development. *Annals of the New York Academy of Sciences, 1094*(1), 13–27. doi:10.1196/annals.1376.003

McAllister, M. (2010). Solution-focused nursing: A fitting model for mental health nurses working in a public health paradigm. *Contemporary Nurse, 34*, 149–157. doi:10.5172/conu.2010.34.2.149

McAllister, M., & McKinnon, J. (2008). The importance of teaching and learning resilience in the health disciplines: A critical review of the literature. *Nurse Education Today, 29*, 371–379. doi:10.1016/j.nedt.2008.10.011

McAllister, M., Moyle, W., & Iselin, G. (2006). Solution focused nursing: An evaluation of current practice. *Nurse Education Today, 26*(5), 439–447. doi:10.1016/j. nedt.2005.12.004

Meehan, T., & Robertson, S. (2013). Clinical profile of people referred to mental health nurses under the Mental Health Nurse Incentive Program. *International Journal of Mental Health Nursing, 22*, 384–390. doi:10.1111/j.1447-0349.2012.00885.x

Mittelmark, M. B., & Bauer, G. F. (2017). The meanings of salutogenesis. In M. B. Mittelmark, S. Sagy, M. Eriksson, G. F. Bauer, J. M. Pelikan, B. Lindstrom, & G. A. Espnes (Eds.), *The handbook of salutogenesis* (pp. 7–14). New York, NY: Springer.

NSW Government, Family & Community Services. (2014). *Working with people with chronic and complex health care needs practice package.* Retrieved from http:// www.adhc.nsw.gov.au/__data/assets/file/0003/301782/Working-with-people -with-chronic-and-complex-health-care-needs-Practice-Package.pdf

Stock, E. (2017). Exploring salutogenesis as a concept of health and wellbeing in nurses who thrive professionally. *British Journal of Nursing, 26*(4), 238–241. doi:10.12968/bjon.2017.26.4.238

Ungar, M. (2008). Resilience across cultures. *British Journal of Social Work, 38*(2), 218–235. doi:10.1093/bjsw/bcl343

Ungar, M. (2011). The social ecology of resilience: Addressing contextual and cultural ambiguity of a nascent construct. *American Journal of Orthopsychiatry, 81*(1), 1–17. doi:10.1111/j.1939-0025.2010.01067.x

Van der Kolk, B. A. (2017). This issue: Child abuse and victimization. *Psychiatric Annals, 35*(5), 374–378. doi:10.3928/00485713-20050501-02

Warelow, P., & Edward, K. L. (2007). Caring as a resilient practice in mental health nursing. *International Journal of Mental Health Nursing, 16*(2), 132–135. doi:10.1111/j.1447-0349.2007.00456.x

West, C., Stewart, L., Foster, K., & Usher, K. (2012). The meaning of resilience to persons living with chronic pain: An interpretive qualitative inquiry. *Journal of Clinical Nursing, 21*(9–10), 1284–1292. doi:10.1111/j.1365-2702.2011.04005.x

Wister, A. V., Coatta, K. L., Schuurman, N., Lear, S. A., Rosin, M., & MacKey, D. (2016). A lifecourse model of multimorbidity resilience: Theoretical and research developments. *The International Journal of Aging and Human Development, 82*(4), 290–313. doi:10.1177/0091415016641686

World Health Organization. (2018). Social determinants of health. Retrieved from http://www.who.int/social_determinants/sdh_definition/en

Yi, J. P., Vitaliano, P. P., Smith, R. E., Yi, J. C., & Weinger, K. (2008). The role of resilience on psychological adjustment and physical health in patients with diabetes. *British Journal of Health Psychology, 13*, 311–325. doi:10.1348/135910707X186994

# 8

# Developing Resilience in Individuals, Services, and Systems

Edward Aquin and Katherine Pachkowski

## INTRODUCTION

This chapter explores the challenge of patients who need to cross healthcare borders because they are dealing with multiple healthcare conditions or chronic diseases, and the challenges this creates for nursing staff. In the healthcare context, a border can be understood as the intersection between the various components of health systems, such as medical and mental health services. Each service often has different foci, routines, and treatments. To the uninitiated, these border crossings can be difficult to navigate and can be the source of much stress. Just like traveling in a foreign country, patients who must use numerous health services can become overwhelmed. Their stress can be compounded if culture, geography, and language are barriers to care and this can negatively impact resilience. Similarly, nurses who need to cross these borders can experience stress in understanding how different parts, and people, of the healthcare system operate.

Such a patient traveler may benefit from a guide, and nurses can learn from their example. In urban health services, this role is increasingly being filled by nurse navigators (Wilcox & Bruce, 2010). At times and in different contexts, however, formal navigators may not be available. In these cases, it falls to individual clinicians to help the patient understand what to expect of each system and how to actively participate in them. Whether a nurse navigator is present or not, all nurses can help the patient build resilience by providing information, support, and advocacy. Nurses can also help by encouraging patients to establish social networks within these systems, which can become a consistent and familiar resource in an all-too-frequently fragmented and difficult to navigate healthcare system. This chapter considers how nurses can help patients build their capacity for resilience, to better cope with the challenges of complicated and varied health systems. It begins with a story from practice that illustrates the complex terrain over which some patients travel.

## ON THE ROAD TO THERAPY ON A CANADIAN WINTER'S DAY

Verna, a Cree woman in her late 50s, woke up early one morning and looked outside to the gray overcast sky, listened to the whistling and howling wind as it whipped up banks of snow to the front of her house. She thought, "I want to go see that counselor today, but first I hope I can get out my front door." The temperature outside was –30 degrees and the wind chill made it feel like –50.

The First Nations Band Administration Office and Nursing Station were in the center of the reservation, half a kilometer away—at least a half hour walk in these blistering conditions. Undeterred, Verna put on her boots, fur trimmed parka, and moose hide mitts that her mother had made. Pushing open the heavy front door, Verna breathed a sigh of relief to feel soft snow giving way to the icy steps underneath. She said to herself, "Glad I am not snowed in, but I had better watch my step going down as I don't want to fall again."

Verna had lived alone since her relationship with Ron had ended a year earlier. To hurt herself now would mean not just pain and injury, but potentially the loss of her home and independence. Like many other women of her age in the community, Verna was grappling with co-associated lifestyle diseases—also called noncommunicable diseases—including diabetes, kidney dysfunction, and hypertension. Now, however, living a healthy lifestyle, including being alcohol-free and physically active, was very important to Verna. Verna also grappled with a severe mental health problem that had recently been exacerbated.

Verna was a child survivor of physical and sexual abuse that happened during her time at residential school. Indian residential or boarding schools operated from the late 19th century until the 1980s, providing mandatory schooling for First Nations children across Canada (Gone, 2013). Many of the children in these schools experienced psychological, physical, and sexual abuse and the adult survivors continue to experience mental distress that has become known as "residential school syndrome" (Brasfield, 2001). The symptoms include those seen in posttraumatic stress disorder— intrusive memories, flashbacks, and anxiety, as well as avoidance of anything that reminds those affected of the residential school experience and ongoing distress related to cultural loss. It is a shameful reality that in many countries and continents across the world—including Australia, Africa, Europe, Ireland, Japan, and the Americas—children and young people were removed from their families and cultures in the name of assimilation and other racist policies. They were institutionalized and subjected to neglect and abuse leading to long-term negative health and social impacts (Armitage, 1995; Mirga, 1993; Rabson, 1996; Smith, 2007).

Like too many others, Verna's childhood involved family separation, hard physical unpaid work, corporal punishment for minor rule infringement, and forbidding cultural practices such as eating traditional foods, smoking rituals, and even speaking the Cree language (Dionne & Nixon, 2013). As an adult, Verna looks back on that time with sadness and anger. More recently, Verna had read about a new government compensation plan for survivors such as herself and, paradoxically, this resulted in a worsening of her trauma and its effects. Verna began having nightmares, panic attacks, and flashbacks. Talking to a qualified mental health worker had been helpful in the past but, because of the remote location in which she lived, clinicians often did not remain long in the area, and so Verna did not know if she would meet a nurse that she would like and trust. A decade ago, mental health workers used to travel twice a month to the community and she could easily attend appointments at the Nursing Station down the road in her community. However, changes to the healthcare funding and governance in local health authorities saw a reduction, rather than an increase, in specialized services to her community. This meant that, in order to attend specialist medical appointments, she needed to travel to a clinic more than 200 km away. To get there, she needed to book the local community bus, or rely on a member of her family to drive her there. In the winter, the roads were often treacherous.

Having reached the local Band Office without slipping or other mishap, Verna was greeted by several familiar faces from her community and the noisy rumble of chesty coughs and babies crying. The visit provided her with a chance to socialize, pick up her pension check, and shop at the local store.

Next, she boarded the community bus and arrived at her scheduled medical appointment without incident in the icy conditions. Usually the clinic arranged for Verna to see a practice nurse who would check her physical status, including her blood pressure and blood sugar, conduct a urine test, and assess any changes in her needs for home-based support. That day, however, Verna was not most concerned about having these tests conducted. She wanted a longer appointment to see the mental health nurse to see what could be done about her sleeplessness and the worries she was feeling. The receptionist then advised Verna that she would need to fill in a number of forms in order to make such a request. This was frustrating, and Verna was also upset to learn that the visiting mental health nurse was running late and that she would need to wait at least an hour to see him. She also began to dread talking to him because she had only met him once before and feared that he would not remember her story, and she would have to repeat it all again.

## THE FRAGMENTED LANDSCAPE OF HEALTHCARE

While "healthcare" is often spoken of as a single, coherent system, fragmentation is a feature of modern health systems (Carter et al., 2018), and creates a host of challenges for both providers and patients. The definition of healthcare fragmentation is when the care a patient needs for an issue must be accessed from two or more different services (Stulberg, Dahlquist, Jarosch, & Lindau, 2016), or when healthcare providers focus on providing care for discrete "parts" of the patient at a time, neglecting the whole (Stange, 2009). Fragmentation also exists when patients move between primary (prevention, first response, and general practice), secondary (treatment centers), and tertiary (rehabilitation and palliative) levels of care, or between different providers, different organizations, or different professionals (Pless, Dessers, & Van Hootegem, 2015). While fragmentation is experienced in different ways, a unifying theme is the notion that healthcare systems are composed of many different pieces that operate independently of one another, but involve movement of patients between them. Sometimes the impact of fragmentation can involve care that is shared between, or distributed across, a number of services. For example, a patient with a respiratory condition may be sent for tests by a general practitioner, referred to a respiratory physician for more tests, and then to a surgeon for a lobectomy. Or, a patient could have a condition that is inadequately treated by one clinician and thus requires the input of numerous service providers. For example, a patient with chronic pain may require a medical specialist to prescribe analgesia, a psychologist to encourage cognitive coping strategies, and a physiotherapist to provide exercise therapy and electrical stimulation treatment.

*Fragmented healthcare delivery can create stress and anxiety in patients, exacerbating vulnerability and increasing risk of treatment nonadherence.*

The way healthcare is funded in various countries also contributes to complexity and fragmentation of care. This is especially true when two or more funding systems are in place in one jurisdiction. In the UK and Australia, for example, some health services run as a public–private partnership, and services and fees are therefore shared. The United States has a vast network of healthcare institutions that are paid for by individuals, insurance agencies (health maintenance organizations), or government agencies (Medicare and Medicaid). In Canada, healthcare in indigenous communities is often funded by the federal government, and healthcare is otherwise provincially delivered (Smylie & Firestone, 2016).

In Verna's case this might mean that her mental healthcare may be covered by federal funding, but the mental health nurse may be an employee of the provincial government or working on contract.

Verna's physical healthcare needs may be covered by provincial funds and communication and coordination between the two bodies may not be streamlined. In general, the system in Canada has been long criticized for being overly complex and riddled with gaps. The flaws in this system are often viewed as a major contributor to the health inequities experienced by indigenous persons in Canada (Smylie & Firestone, 2016).

Fragmentation provides challenges to healthcare providers and patients. While compartmentalization is a pragmatic necessity in today's specialized healthcare world, levels of disconnection exist among the different healthcare services, and it is often left to the patient to navigate these different systems alone. In terms of Verna's experience, she has a history that is deeply personal as well as cultural, and the stressors she is experiencing as a result are ongoing. She has physical health challenges that require different medical specialists. Her remote location comes with its own challenges, including the physical difficulty of accessing services far from home, and not experiencing a continuity of care as many staff come and go from the services she uses. Verna's distress is understandable, yet her strength in persisting with care is admirable. Many patients in Verna's situation do not adhere to the treatments that are available to them, and which they need.

Healthcare fragmentation can lead to poor health outcomes (Everson, Adler-Milstein, Hollingsworth, & Shoou-Yih Daniel, 2017) and low patient satisfaction (Stange, 2009). Fragmentation means that patients and healthcare providers may struggle to communicate and coordinate care among different services. Poor coordination leads to miscommunication and feelings of frustration for the different clinical providers and this is subtly yet powerfully conveyed to patients, who mirror their clinicians' feelings of confusion and frustration (Stange, 2009). Additionally, when clinicians are not supplied with sufficient health histories or other information they require from clinical colleagues in other specialties, the risks that patients receive inadequate or inappropriate treatments rise. These risks multiply when these patients are from marginalized cultural backgrounds. Research and experience confirm that patients from culturally and linguistically diverse backgrounds frequently experience many challenges in this process: They may feel patronized, excluded, or controlled; fail to understand which service to access and how; not know how to transition among different types of care; and feel ill-equipped to deal with inappropriate care (Carter et al., 2018). Consequently, they often feel overwhelmed confused, anxious, and unsatisfied.

*Continuity of care, facilitated by nurse navigators and clear communication among the clinical team, improves patient outcomes.*

On the other hand, however, when there is strong continuity of care among the different systems, patients' health outcomes are improved, and hospital length of stay and readmission rates are reduced (Ahuja & Staats, 2017). Interprofessional understanding also improves communication and complete care (Zwarenstein, Goldman, & Reeves, 2009). Improvements are also seen when health practitioners have a continuous relationship with patients because familiarity, trust, and open communication often flow (Guthrie, Saultz, Freeman, & Haggerty, 2008). This is also, obviously, more satisfying and less stressful for nurses and the other healthcare providers involved in such unfragmented care.

## STRATEGIES TO BUILD RESILIENCE

Nurses can work in practical ways to assist patients to navigate and safely cross healthcare borders and, in the process, build their resilience, maximizing their strengths and motivation to achieve goals, to engage with care, and to maintain their healthy progress. Patients can be empowered through numerous inspiring and motivating actions, including open dialogue, targeted educational discussions, and interventions, and the development of social networks, providing advocacy and supporting a patient's self-advocacy. The development and support of the nurse navigator role is another contributor to patient empowerment.

### Communication and Education

If patients do not understand the healthcare system, they are more likely to be passive recipients of care, or avoidant and fail to access care in timely ways (Carter et al., 2018). Therefore, nurses who generally hold a trusted position by virtue of their close relationship with patients, have the potential to make a real difference in educating patients. This can be achieved directly during conversations with patients. In this dialogue, it is important that nurses use language that is familiar and understandable to their patients, and to regularly check in with these patients to ensure they understand the issues and the consequences of choices. In dialogue with the patient, nurses can explore the patient's internal resources, strengths, and resilience, and learn more about any available external resources and support networks. During such interactions, nurses can gain a better understanding of the patient's current understanding of the healthcare system and can help reduce ambiguity and misunderstandings. Nurses must also respect their patients' autonomy. This means respecting their capacities to decide what is best for themselves. At times, it means respecting that patients' individual, cultural, or community context may lead to informed decisions with which the nurse may not agree.

Nurses can also provide education in ways that are less direct but can reach many, and stimulate new thinking and transformed perspectives about health, illness, and recovery. Use of culturally relevant posters, podcasts, comics, television and Internet advertisements, radio broadcasts and shopping center displays are examples.

## Social Support Networks

Patients who have well-developed social support networks are better able to successfully navigate complex healthcare systems and are more likely to restore and sustain mental health and well-being. Knowing this, carers often take on the role of informal service navigators (Olasoji, Maude, & McCauley, 2017). They are well positioned to recognize when a patient's well-being is suffering or their health is deteriorating (Olasoji et al., 2017). They can also approach friends and peers to share their experiences and provide recommendations and guidance. Communities or families can also come together to provide practical support. In communities like Verna's, for example, it is common for community members to help each other with transportation to healthcare clinics. Family members can attend appointments with patients and help them process information. They can also, invaluably, provide patients with motivation and inspiration to continue to take the necessary actions to improve their health.

While not an ideal situation, caregivers of people with an illness often take on the role of coordinator of care (Happell, Wilson, Platania-Phung, & Stanton, 2016). Caregivers and other support persons can help patients navigate the fragmented healthcare system. Nurses should therefore include these support persons in their educational activities, but should also be mindful of the burden of care that family members might be required to take on (Olasoji et al., 2017). The nurse may consider recommending and taking possible actions that might alleviate the burdens and stressors on caregivers.

## Advocacy

Nurses have power within the healthcare system and can use that power to advocate for change on behalf of their patients. Nurses can advocate for policy change that increases communication and coordination across healthcare systems. In addition, nurses can advocate for patients on a personal level as they attempt to make contact with other service providers.

Self-advocacy is the ability to effectively communicate one's desires and needs and is interdependent with self-determination (Paradiz, Kelso, Nelson, & Earl, 2018). It is a powerful tool that can help patients and their families receive care from different systems as needed. As with resilience, self-advocacy can be taught and nurtured. Nurses can encourage self-advocacy by, for example, providing opportunities for patients to practice what it is they want to ask for, or say to, other clinicians. The nurse can provide feedback to and coach patients, helping them to be prepared, articulate, and persistent. It is also important for nurses to recognize when a patient is being a self-advocate and respect that patient's wishes accordingly, rather than mislabeling that patient as difficult or noncompliant.

## Nurse Navigators

Longstanding global concerns have been expressed by the World Health Organization (2015) about inequitable access to healthcare services based on geography and socioeconomic conditions. Over the past two decades, advancements have been made as a result of research and the development of service navigation roles in healthcare environments. The concept of health service navigation emerged in oncology (Freeman, 2013). Because cancer care often takes place over an extended period, involving the use of many services, the navigator role was developed to help patients find their way through these services and their providers and feel less anxious. They also ensure that the various services communicate well with the patient, passing on information in a timely way so that the patient understands this and does not receive inappropriate care.

Over time, nurse navigator roles have begun to develop in other areas of health such as emergency departments (Jessup, Fulbrook, & Kinnear, 2017) and community primary care roles (Carter et al., 2018). These roles have emerged in countries such as the United States, Canada, and Australia. Irrespective of the health service environment, the primary role of a nurse navigator is to assist individuals and their families to overcome gaps in the healthcare system, and ultimately to improve the health literacy and health outcomes of patients (McMurray & Cooper, 2017). When formal nurse navigator roles are absent, nurses working in any setting should remember that service integration and ease of transition should be the goal for all patients. Because nurses have a broad skill base, involving familiarity with medical terms and treatments and a value-base that involves cultural sensitivity, social justice, and patient empowerment, they are well placed to provide this service navigation. Done well, the nurse navigator role—whether performed formally or informally—improves social integration, reduces service barriers, and connects patients to health and social services (Feather, Carter, Valaitas, & Kirkpatrick, 2017).

The following story provides insight into this navigator role, from the perspective of Mark, the mental health nurse who provided care for Verna. As you will read, Mark's role was a diverse one and his aim was to bridge numerous healthcare borders to facilitate safe and comprehensive collaborative care for Verna.

## OWÎCIHTÂSIW: ONE WHO IS A HELPER OF PEOPLE

On the same day that Verna made her way to the clinic, Mark, a senior mental health nurse, made his way to work from his cabin on the lake. Mark loved his lifestyle in this remote place; the scenery of boreal forest, the colors of the trees in autumn, the winter sports such as snowmobiling and ice fishing. These activities are, however, a rarity for the nurse as he spends many hours trying to keep on top of the paperwork from his excessive workload. As a mental health clinician, he has more than 80 patients on his caseload, ranging from single session crisis intakes to chronic care patients that have been on the caseload for years. Despite the challenges and expectations of the role, Mark is committed to service provision and to the community he serves.

Mark is from a "White" English-speaking farming background and faced a steep learning curve when he moved to the blended "White" and First Nations community. He had to bridge a cultural divide when providing services. In this case, he found he had to allow time for verbal responses, adjust his level of eye contact, and build his awareness of First Nations traditional healing practices. He often worked with individuals who spoke French or Cree as their first language. When initially trying to introduce himself during assessments as a mental health nurse, he was met by comments such as "I'm not mental" or "I don't want to see a mental nurse." He realized that some people held biases about mental health and mental health nurses that could be a serious barrier to care. Mark decided to consult an elder about the issue. The elder advised Mark to change his clinical title to a Cree term for a social worker or helper: Owîcihtâsiw. Unpronounceable to Mark, though meaningful to many Cree patients, he settled on verbally introducing himself to people as "a professional helper."

Over the years, mental health services to remote communities such as the one Verna lives in, have been reduced in a cost-saving effort. As a result, the services provided for clients such as Verna were limited to tele-health and monthly mental health visiting services. In planning for his day as Mark neared town, he recalled that there was an intake meeting with his supervisor and team. Intake meetings discuss all new patient referrals and their expected needs. Mark knew this would take most of the morning and he needed to be prepared for his afternoon patients. He knew that his first scheduled patient was Verna, and Mark remembered Verna well—a survivor of childhood abuse, family violence, and a feisty funny lady, who he instantly admired.

While waiting for the meeting to start, Mark emailed Verna's primary care clinician to ensure that she had follow-up appointments with the diabetes educator, and to ensure that the family doctor has completed new prescriptions so that she could collect them later that day. His preparations completed, Mark was then notified that two of the mental health team would not be attending because of the weather conditions, and that he would therefore have to take all the intake calls for the day, as well as see his regular patients. He also learned that a new funding stream had been established by the federal government for private providers to provide therapy services for individuals affected by residential school trauma. This meant that he would not be permitted to provide ongoing care for Verna and, more than likely, her future counseling would have to be provided via tele-health. He had a feeling that Verna would not like this new arrangement and began to feel anxious about their interaction later that day.

Mark suggested to the team that this change should not be accepted without protest. He argued that patients affected by residential school syndrome were particularly vulnerable and required culturally sensitive, face-to-face care as well as delicate handling in order to facilitate safe handovers from one clinician to the next. Mark proposed that they should write to the policy provider suggesting a partnership be developed between the federally funded First Nations health services, the provincial service, and the local indigenous community. Although this was not a formal nurse navigator arrangement, the connection of services for patients would likely be welcomed and achieve positive health outcomes. Just as Mark finished explaining his innovative model, the phone rang, and he was asked to see a patient who had presented in crisis and needed to be seen immediately. It was almost an hour later until he was able, finally, to meet with Verna.

## How Mark Fosters Resilience

Mark's story provides an opportunity to evaluate actions and practices that foster resilience in the face of challenges working in, and across, numerous health borders. Mark was posted to a remote service far removed from friends and family, but he promoted his own resilience by connecting to the local community and enjoying the sports and culture. This helped him establish a sense of belonging, identity, and understanding of the environment so he could adapt to life in this remote environment. Mark also practiced nursing in a way that targeted political and public policy action as well as personal, patient-centered actions that navigated a person's movement safely across numerous borders. He began his posting with little knowledge of Cree culture and, realizing this, sought out an elder to expand his cultural knowledge and acceptance. He exercised creative, political problem-solving when faced with the challenge of service cuts and harm to patients, by suggesting a new model of care. Mark also worked to promote Verna's resilience by ensuring—in the short time that they had together—that the services she needed were available to her. In summary, Mark implemented psychological, social, and structural strengths. The psychological strengths included cognitive problem-solving. The social strengths he demonstrated included seeking support, demonstrating empathy for others, and acting to do good in the workplace for both his and other patients. His structural strengths included seeing health inequities as requiring political solutions and a willingness to work to initiate policy change.

## CONCLUSION

Healthcare fragmentation is a common feature of contemporary healthcare systems. As a patient moves among different services, levels of care, and various providers, they are likely to experience challenges and frustration. Nurses can help patients navigate these systems. All nurses can help patients learn what to expect from the different services available that they are likely to encounter. Instead of feeling powerless or frustrated themselves, nurses can both help encourage self-advocacy in their patients at a personal and practical level, and advocate for patients' needs and preferences at the political level. Assisting patients in this way as they move among parts of the healthcare system will ensure better health outcomes and greater patient satisfaction, as well as less frustration and more occupational fulfillment for nurses and other healthcare staff.

## LEARNING ACTIVITIES

1. Thinking about the resilience standpoint elaborated on in earlier chapters, identify the psychological, social, cultural, and structural resources that are present or absent in Verna's story.

2. Suggest what immediate actions the mental health nurse could have taken in order to empathize, and engage, with Verna.

3. *IMAGINE A CANADA: Celebrating Youth Visions for Reconciliation* (National Centre for Truth and Reconciliation, 2017) is a webbook that illustrates school children's dreams of the future for indigenous peoples of Canada. Please follow this link to view the illustrations: https://education.nctr.ca/wp-content/uploads/2018/02/2017-NCTR-IMAGINE-A-CANADA-WEBBOOK.pdf

   • What is the Truth and Reconciliation Commission (TRC) of Canada's mandate and how does the TRC support survivors of residential schools?
   • How do the narratives by survivors told to the younger generation in their schools promote healing, cultural identity and resilience?
   • What benefits do you see about this initiative that could apply to other cultures that have been marginalized and experienced intergenerational loss and grief.

4. Identify and appraise the expanded scope of practice that Nurse Navigators undertake in a primary healthcare setting.

5. If Canadian: Define and differentiate the symptoms of posttraumatic stress disorder and residential school syndrome. Compare and evaluate treatment interventions found in contemporary literature that promote resilience from a cultural perspective.

6. If from a country other than Canada: Compare and evaluate treatment interventions found in contemporary literature that promote resilience from the cultural perspectives of your own country.

## REFERENCES

Ahuja, V., & Staats, B. R. (2017). *Continuity in gatekeepers: Quantifying the impact of care fragmentation.* SMU Cox School of Business Research Paper No. 18-17. Retrieved from https://ssrn.com/abstract=3091130 or http://dx.doi.org/10.2139/ssrn.3091130

Armitage, A. (1995). *Comparing the policy of aboriginal assimilation: Australia, Canada, and New Zealand.* Vancouver, Canada: UBC Press.

Brasfield, C. (2001). Residential school syndrome. *BC Medical Journal, 43*(2), 78–81.

Carter, N., Valaitis, R. K., Lam, A., Feather, J., Nicholl, J., & Cleghorn, L. (2018). Navigation delivery models and roles of navigators in primary care: A scoping literature review. *BMC Health Services Research, 18*, 1–13. doi:10.1186/s12913-018-2889-0

Dionne, D., & Nixon, G. (2013). Moving beyond residential school trauma abuse: A phenomenological hermeneutic analysis. *International Journal of Mental Health and Addiction, 12*, 335–350. doi:10.1007/s11469-013-9457-y

Everson, J., Adler-Milstein, J., Hollingsworth, J., & Shoou-Yih Daniel, L. (2017). A network approach to care fragmentation: Impact on the quality and efficiency of hospital care. *Academy of Management Annual Meeting Proceedings, 2017*(1), 16183. doi:10.5465/AMBPP.2017.16183abstract

Feather, J., Carter, N., Valaitas, R., & Kirkpatrick, H. (2017). A narrative evaluation of a community-based navigation role in an urban at-risk community. *Journal of Advanced Nursing, 73*, 2997–3006. doi:10.1111/jan.13355

Freeman, H. (2013). The history, principles, and future of patient navigation: Commentary. *Seminars in Oncology Nursing, 29*(2), 72–75. doi:10.1016/j.soncn.2013.02.002

Gone, P. J. (2013). Redressing First Nations historical trauma: Theorizing mechanisms for indigenous culture as mental health treatment. *Transcultural Psychiatry, 50*(5), 683–706. doi:10.1177/1363461513487669

Guthrie, B., Saultz, J. W., Freeman, G. K., & Haggerty, J. L. (2008). Continuity of care matters. *BMJ: British Medical Journal (Online), 337*, a867.

Happell, B., Wilson, K., Platania-Phung, C., & Stanton, R. (2016). Filling the gaps and finding our way: Family carers navigating the healthcare system to access physical health services for the people they care for. *Journal of Clinical Nursing, 16*, 1917–1926.

Jessup, M., Fulbrook, P., & Kinnear, F. (2017). Multidisciplinary evaluation of an emergency department nurse navigator role: A mixed methods study. *Australian Critical Care, 31*(5), 303–310. doi:10.1016/j.aucc.2017.08.006

McMurray, A., & Cooper, H. (2017). The nurse navigator: An evolving model of care. *Collegian, 24*, 205–212. doi:10.1016/j.colegn.2016.01.002

Mirga, A. (1993). The effects of state assimilation policy on Polish gypsies. *Romani Studies, 3*(2), 69.

National Centre for Truth and Reconciliation. (2017). *Imagine a Canada: Celebrating youth visions for reconciliation.* Winnipeg, MB, Canada: Author. Retrieved from https://education.nctr.ca/wp-content/uploads/2018/02/2017-NCTR-IMAGINE-A-CANADA-WEBBOOK.pdf

Olasoji, M., Maude, P., & McCauley, K. (2017). Not sick enough: Experiences of carers of people with mental illness negotiating care for their relatives with mental health services. *Journal of Psychiatric & Mental Health Nursing, 24*(6), 403–411. doi:10.1111/jpm.12399

Paradiz, V., Kelso, S., Nelson, A., & Earl, A. (2018). Essential self-advocacy and transition. *Pediatrics, 141*(Suppl. 4), S373–S377. doi:10.1542/peds.2016-4300P

Pless, S., Dessers, E., & Van Hootegem, G. (2015). Mapping care fragmentation in terms of task division. *International Journal of Integrated Care, 15*, 19–21. Retrieved from https://dspace.library.uu.nl/handle/1874/323375

Rabson, S. (1996). *Assimilation policy in Okinawa: Promotion, resistance and "reconstruction."* Japan Policy Research Institute. Occasional Paper. Retrieved from http://www.jpri.org/publications/occasionalpapers/op8.html

Smith, J. (2007). *Magdalen laundries and the nation's architect of containment.* Notre Dame, IN: University of the Notre Dame Press.

Smylie, J., & Firestone, M. (2016). The health of indigenous peoples. In D. Rafael (Ed.), *Social determinants of health: Canadian perspectives* (3rd ed., pp. 434–466). Toronto, ON, Canada: Canadian Scholars Press.

Stange, K. C. (2009). The problem of fragmentation and the need for integrative solutions. *Annals of Family Medicine, 7*(2), 100–103. doi:10.1370/afm.971

Stulberg, D., Dahlquist, I., Jarosch, C., & Lindau, S. (2016). Fragmentation of care in ectopic pregnancy. *Maternal & Child Health Journal, 20*(5), 955–961. doi:10.1007/s10995-016-1979-z

Wilcox, B., & Bruce, S. (2010). Patient navigation: A "win-win" for all involved. *Oncology Nursing Forum, 37*(1), 21. doi:10.1188/10.ONF.21-25

World Health Organization. (2015). *Health workforce and services: Draft global strategy on human resources for health: Workforce 2030* (Executive Board 138th session Provisional agenda item 10.1 EB 138/36) Retrieved from http://apps.who.int/iris/bitstream/handle/10665/250703/B138_36- en.pdf?sequence=1&isAllowed=y

Zwarenstein, M., Goldman, J., & Reeves, S. (2009). Interprofessional collaboration: Effects of practice-based interventions on professional practice and healthcare outcomes. *Cochrane Database of Systemic Reviews, 8*(3), 1–30. doi:10.1002/14651858. CD000072.pub2

# 9

# Activating Resilience Under Stress

Sherry S. Chesak and Susanne Cutshall

## INTRODUCTION

By now readers will appreciate the multiple sources of occupational stress in nursing—being close to people in distress and crisis is stressful, as are the demands of the work. Nursing involves rotating shifts, heavy workloads and time pressures in the care of the patients with complex, ever-changing healthcare needs. The hazards of nursing for nurses can also include physical injury, infections, needle sticks, and chemical exposures. Finally, the demands of the role can have a negative impact on the mental health of nurses, who are at greater risk for depression and burnout than the general population (Brandford & Reed, 2016). In addition to these factors, the increased rate of mental health and drug and alcohol issues impacting patients' health lead to a high likelihood of nurses experiencing traumatic events in the workplace (Pekurinen et al., 2017).

The purpose of this chapter is to identify the extreme adversity that nurses face globally on a daily basis, which impacts their ability to cope and maintain their health and well-being. At times, the challenges can seem overwhelming and even insurmountable, which has the potential to lead nurses to leave the profession. However, there are measures that nurses can take to manage stress pre-emptively, in the moment that it is occurring, and after traumatic events; measures that will allow them to cope with adversity, and to come out of adversity a stronger individual and a healthier, more effective nurse. Healthcare systems and nursing organizations also have an obligation to improve the nursing work environment and identify measures that are effective in mitigating adverse events that negatively impact the well-being of nurses and the care that they provide.

The following scenarios portray the personal stories of two nurses who have experienced traumatic events in the workplace. In the first story, Amanda was new to the profession and experienced her first challenging event. She has not yet developed skills to assist her with coping with such an event and therefore becomes overwhelmed by the situation and finds herself questioning her choice of profession. In the second story, Kristin is an experienced nurse who has developed coping skills that improve her resilience and allow her to stay strong in the face of adversity. The stories demonstrate the fact that resilience is not necessarily inherent; however, with experience, and practicing the principles that build resilience, nurses can adjust more positively to adversity.

## AMANDA'S STORY

Amanda graduated from a nursing program 3 months ago and is settling into her first job as an RN in the emergency department of a large metropolitan hospital. She is excited about her new role as a professional nurse and is gradually adjusting to many changes in her life. She has also just moved to the big city from her small college town and is living on her own for the first time. This means, however, that she is not only busy navigating the responsibilities that come with the new role, but those associated with the move as well. She has just recently completed her orientation at the hospital and is feeling confident that she is prepared to practice independently as a nurse.

On the day that this story revolves around, she arrived at the hospital for her 12-hour night shift, and received report from the evening shift. She learned that it was a relatively standard day in the emergency department, with the usual business of patients coming and going. Shortly after her shift began, she was called to assist with a patient who she was advised was experiencing delirium. She arrived to find an elderly man in the corner of the patient room with his walker up over the top of his head, yelling, "If anyone comes near me, I will hit you." Amanda quickly drew on what she learned during her studies about de-escalating agitated patients. Although a security officer showed up in the door, she asked him to leave as she did not want him to agitate the patient more. Another nurse came to the door and told Amanda that they had looked up the patient's history and he was a war veteran who suffers from posttraumatic stress disorder (PTSD). He had received an initial diagnosis, which could be treated, but he could not afford psychological or pharmacological treatments. Amanda decided that the best first course of action was to start an IV on the patient, anticipating that the provider would order an antipsychotic medication that will act quickly and help to temper his agitation. She told the patient that she was not going to hurt him, but needed to have him lay in the bed so she could help him. She slowly walked toward the patient, but he swung the walker at her, hitting her and causing her to fall to the floor and injure her wrist. The patient then lost his balance, and also fell to the floor, suffering a fracture to his skull, and was then transferred to the intensive care unit. Amanda found her own wrist was fractured, requiring her to take leave from work. Upon her return, she learnt that a couple of days after this event, the patient had died.

Upon learning this, Amanda felt completely distraught and questioned what she could have done differently to manage the situation. She felt largely responsible for the patient's death and it weighed on her heavily. She questioned a healthcare system that would allow a patient to go untreated for a mental illness that most likely led to his death. She also began to experience panic attacks when called to assist with similar situations.

Less than 1 year into her nursing career, Amanda has become uncomfortable sharing concerns with colleagues as she does not want to give the impression that she cannot handle her job. She has also begun to wonder whether nursing is the right profession for her if all of this is part of the job.

Amanda is not alone in her experience of patient aggression and the consequent negative effects on nurses' well-being. Working in the emergency department or psychiatric unit are the two most likely sites of patient-initiated violence (Pekurinen et al., 2017). That Amanda does not feel safe in disclosing concerns or asking for support from colleagues only places her more at risk for the accumulation of stressors that may eventually lead to her own development of trauma, an inability to effectively care for others.

While many nurses are unprepared for patient-initiated violence, there are also those who have trained especially for this consequence, and in Kristin's story, a very different outcome is achieved, such that this nurse not only survives a challenging encounter, but feels a sense of efficacy and collegial connection that make her more likely to continue to care for others compassionately and effectively.

## KRISTIN'S STORY

Kristin has been a nurse for 17 years. She began her career on a general medical/surgical floor in a rural hospital where she learned a wide range of nursing skills. After 5 years of experience, she noted that she was particularly skilled at assisting patients with mental health issues and therefore decided to take a position in the inpatient behavioral health unit at the same hospital. After working in the role for a couple of years, Kristin decided to continue to advance her skills in working with patients with psychiatric and behavioral issues and took a job with the behavioral emergency response team (BERT). The BERT team was a multidisciplinary team that responds to behavioral patient issues and provides guidance on interventions and resources individualized to each situation. Kristin enjoyed this position and, after many years of experience in the role, her skills advanced and she became an expert nurse who many members of the healthcare team relied on for her expertise in behavioral health issues. She had also learned the importance of taking care of herself through proper nutrition, sleep, and exercise so that she could be present for her patients and skillfully care for them. She has also found that mindfulness practices helped her de-stress at the end of each busy work day.

One evening on the job she was paged to the behavioral health unit as staff there had been managing a patient with borderline personality disorder who had gotten hold of a knife and was threatening to harm herself. Kristin had received a report on the patient at the start of the shift and knew that she had wanted to go home that day, but the provider had told her that she could not leave. When Kristin arrived, the knife had been removed, but she was now pounding on the bed loudly and demanding to be released. Kristin noted the room was dark and turned on the lights in an attempt to reorient the patient. She called the patient by name, and calmly stated, "Cindy, I am not going to hurt you, are you going to hurt me?" The patient replied, "What do you want from me?" Kristin let the patient know she just wanted to talk to her, and then reminded her of where she was and what day it was. Cindy seemed to calm down slightly, but remained upset and told Kristin that she just wanted to get out because no one was helping her. Kristin identified with the patient's frustrations and stated "Cindy, you are very upset because you are being asked to stay in the hospital, but you don't feel like anyone is helping you here. I understand that you would be frustrated about that. I would like to help you, do you want my help?" The patient calmed down further and replied that she did. Kristin then told Cindy that she understood that she was upset, but she needed to find a way to let out her frustrations without disturbing the other patients on the unit. The patient proceeded to let off energy by pounding on her bed and screaming in her pillow (but without disturbing other patients), and continued the activity for an hour until she eventually calmed down.

At the end of the shift, Kristin debriefed about this patient event with the oncoming BERT nurse, Steve, and they discussed how she handled the situation, what the potential outcomes were, and how she avoided potential negative outcomes. Steve supported Kristin through his attuned listening (sensing and understanding her needs with the purpose of helping her regulate her emotions), cooperative inquiry (collaborating with her to make sense of the situation and develop new and creative ways of managing similar situations in the future), and optimism (providing her with hope for positive outcomes with future traumatic events). As a result, Kristin returned to her home tired from her challenging day, but looking forward to what the next would bring. Before going to bed she practiced a mindful movement exercise to de-stress and help relax her for a refreshing sleep.

Kristin's experience contrasts markedly with that of Amanda's. Her training in aggression management helped her to approach the patient respectfully and nonthreateningly so that trust was gained. Kristin conveyed to the patient an understanding of the sources of tension and also encouraged the safe outlet of that stress. Even so, it must have been a highly emotionally charged encounter, and Kristin sought the support of a colleague who knew how to be empathetic, to facilitate catharsis of any pent-up anxiety, and to encourage self-compassion and a positive outlook for the future. She also incorporated a practice of mindfulness in her daily life to de-stress and, consequently, be more available to her patients.

## CHALLENGES IN THE WORKPLACE

Contemporary nurses are facing new challenges in the workplace. Violence against nurses is at epidemic levels, yet few studies have addressed the impact of violence on nurses' quality of life and nurses' intention to leave their jobs. In one such study in 2014, it was estimated that three out of every four nurses experience some type of verbal or physical abuses in the workplace (Duncan et al., 2016). This could include yelling, cursing, grabbing, scratching, kicking, or worse and can come from both patients and their visitors.

According to a study by Speroni, Fitch, Dawson, Dugan, and Atherton (2014) conducted at a U.S. urban/community hospital system with over 5,000 nurses, of the 762 nurses that responded to a survey, 76% had experienced violence over the past year. Emergency nurses experienced a significantly greater number of incidents. In this facility, the perpetrators of this violence were primarily White males, aged 26 to 35 years, who were confused or influenced by alcohol or drugs. A study in Korea by Choi and Lee (2017) found that of 358 nurses surveyed, 95.5% had experienced workplace violence over the previous year. According to the U.S. Centers for Disease Control and Prevention (CDC), between 2012 and 2014, nurses and nursing assistants experienced higher workplace violence injuries than other healthcare workers (CDC, 2015).

Most healthcare providers adjust well to the multitude of demands encountered during an unexpected or traumatic clinical event, and often have strong emotional defenses that carry them through and let them "get the job done." Yet sometimes the emotional aftershock (or stress reaction) can be difficult. Signs and symptoms of this emotional aftershock may last a few days, a few weeks, a few months, or longer. This is called second victim's phenomenon (Seys et al., 2013), and occurs when healthcare workers experience significant stress, violence, or distress. Second victims are "healthcare providers who are involved in an unanticipated adverse patient event, medical error and/or a patient related injury and become victimized in the sense that the provider is traumatized by the event" (Scott et al., 2010, p. 233). If those in the profession do not come to second victims' aid in times of need, these second victims may suffer sleepless nights, burnout, or other impacts that can harm their ability to provide care that is compassionate, high quality, and safe.

*The suffering of caregivers in the face of a serious medical problem has been termed second victim's phenomenon.*

## CREATIVE RESPONSES TO PREVENT CAREGIVER TRAUMA

This care to staff needs to be timely because, most of the time, caregivers are pressed back into service quickly after a traumatic event. There are more patients needing their help, a busy schedule, and colleagues who depend on them to get through the day. When compelled to go immediately back to work after a traumatic event, memories and feelings surrounding the event can be repressed— pushed out of conscious awareness—only to emerge later in how these caregivers react at work and home or to changes (Gates, Gillespie, & Succop, 2011). Some institutions have recognized the importance of responding with debriefing during these times (Quillivan, Burlison, Browne, Scott, & Hoffman, 2016) and a growing number of studies have emphasized the need for organizational emotional support programs to be provided for healthcare workers (Allen & Palk, 2018; Grawitch, Gottschalk, & Munz, 2006; Van Gerven et al., 2016).

The American Nurses Association (ANA) has recognized that nurses are experiencing work and life stressors that not only affect them but also their ability to be of support to their patients and thus the health of the nation in which they work. Key findings of the ANA's health risk appraisal show that the health of American nurses is often worse than that of the average American. Nurses are often overweight, get less sleep, and have higher levels of stress than the average American. Hazards such as workplace violence contribute to their poorer health. A similar situation has been identified with Australian nurses (Happell et al., 2013).

As a result, the ANA supports the Nurse's Bill of Rights that includes a statement that nurses have the right to a work environment that is safe for themselves and their patients. The ANA has also started a campaign entitled *Healthy Nurse, Healthy Grand Challenge Program* as a nationwide movement to connect and engage nurses and organizations to take positive action in physical activity, sleep, nutrition, quality of life, and safety (ANA, 2018). This includes providing access to resources, webinars, newsletters, well-being challenges, and ways to connect with other nurses. Effective workplace programs are still needed for wellness, safe patient handling and mobility, needle stick prevention, workplace violence, stress reduction, and other issues. Nurses who are working at the front line of care need to be involved in the planning and implementation of these programs at each stage of their development and implementation.

## STRESS MANAGEMENT INTERVENTIONS FOR NURSES

There is growing interest in identifying stress management interventions for nurses that are effective in improving nurses' mental health and well-being and the quality of care they provide, as well as in an effort to attract and retain nursing staff. Interventions that have been studied can be divided into three categories: those aimed at treatment of the individual, those aimed at treatment of the work environment, and those that combine both methods (Romppanen & Häggman-Laitila, 2017). The preponderance of the current evidence is related to interventions aimed at treatment of the individual, leaving a gap in knowledge on which types of interventions aimed at the environment are most effective.

A wide variety of interventions aimed at the individual have been tested including mindfulness-based interventions, psychological skills training, coping and support groups, massage, energy therapies, yoga, and other physical activity training. Due to the lack of large-scale, well-designed, randomized controlled trials, it is difficult to synthesize the literature and determine best practices for reducing nurse stress. It is evident, however, that long-term stress management interventions that include refresher sessions have proven most effective (Romppanen & Häggman-Laitila, 2017). It is important for nurse leaders to be aware of these interventions and to support staff in pursuing a variety of activities.

## The Brain and Stress

The brain is a complex organ that is made up of an intricate system of billions of neurons that connect to make networks. Having a better understanding of how the brain works, and how it operates when under stress, can assist with identifying the practices that contribute to managing stress and building resilience. Amit Sood of the Mayo Clinic describes two main modes of the brain: the focused mode and the default mode (Sood, 2013). The focused mode is engaged when we are intentionally focusing on an experience or are occupied with purposeful thoughts. The default mode, on the other hand, is activated when the mind is wandering, ruminating, or caught in automatic, internally directed thinking. Often, these thoughts are biased to be neutral or negative. Human brains are hardwired to escape the present moment and engage in the default network. This leads to a focus on fears, regrets, and wants, which generates stress, weakens attention, and causes internal conflict. However, attention training—where one is intentional about one's presence—can lead to more time spent in the focused mode and more effective stress management and resilience.

*Interventions that train the mind to focus on positive aspects of the present moment appear to prevent lapsing into rumination and worry that exacerbates stress.*

Dr. Sood's Stress Management and Resiliency Training (SMART) program is now used both nationally in the United States and internationally as a simple, flexible approach to incorporate attention training principles into daily life. The practices included in the program serve to pull the thinker into an intentional presence, and thus experience more joy and compassion (focused mode), versus automatic focus on regrets in the past or fears for the future (default mode). At the core of the program are practices that assist with reclaiming attention and focusing intentionally, such as paying attention to novelty in everyday life (viewing things through the eyes of a child, for instance, or immersing oneself in nature and noting the novelty of a single flower). Other practices in the program include methods to cultivate a resilient mindset through focusing on gratitude, acceptance, meaning-making, forgiveness, and compassion—principles that research has shown effectively reduce stress and build resilience (Sood, 2010). Engaging regularly in gratitude practice—ideally by keeping a daily journal to document being thankful for specific things in your life that you are grateful for and appreciate—has shown promise in a number of studies for reducing stress and improving happiness (Kyeong, Kim, Kim, Kim, & Kim, 2017). Acceptance allows one to focus on what is truly important and what one can control versus becoming over-whelmed with circumstances that are out of one's control. Finding meaning in one's work is an important practice that prevents burnout, particularly in healthcare professions (Pines, 2017). The practice of forgiveness also allows one to let go of anger and resentment and choose a higher path that leads to peace and happiness.

Conversely, overwork in the healthcare setting can negatively impact healthcare professionals' ability to engage in self-care, and also detract from the care provided to their patients (Mills, Wand, & Fraser, 2015). Therefore, it is critical that nurses find meaning through building personal and professional relationships (building one's "tribe"), in the work that they do, and through focused mode activities or spiritual practices.

## Compassion

Perhaps the resilience principle that is most aligned and key to nursing practice is that of compassion. Nurses often enter the profession because they have a desire to care for others (Price, 2009). However, providing care for patients with complex issues and in an ever-changing healthcare environment can be draining and, over the years, can lead to burnout. True compassion, on the other hand, is energizing and enhances well-being and happiness. The practice of compassion encompasses decreasing others' suffering through forming meaningful connections with them and transforming their experience. It is not simply feeling sorry for others; rather, it is feeling their suffering with them and taking action to help them to heal and/or cope. According to Sood, compassionate care includes four steps: recognizing others' suffering, validating others' suffering, setting an intention to decrease suffering, and taking action to decrease suffering and sustain compassion even in the face of adversity.

*Practicing compassion, aiming to relieve the suffering of others, gives nurses meaning and a sense of effectiveness in their work.*

## Empathy

The concept of empathy is closely related to compassion and involves the ability to place oneself in someone else's position and see things from his and her perspective. The process of recognizing patients' distress cues and allowing them to open up about their emotional distress has been termed "empathic communication" (Suchman, Markakis, Beckman, & Frankel, 1997), and is a crucial skill for healthcare providers to hone. Silverman, Kurtz, and Draper (1998) define empathy as "a two-stage process: 1) the understanding and sensitive appreciation of another person's predicament or feelings and 2) the communication of that understanding back to the patient in a supportive way" (p. 83). Empathic communication has been demonstrated to improve patient outcomes through two key mechanisms: leading patients to disclose more about their symptoms and concerns, and assisting the patient to feel listened to, valued, understood, and accepted (Neumann et al., 2009).

## Self-Compassion

Self-compassion—showing kindness and empathy to oneself (Neff, 2016)—is an important component of practicing compassion. Practicing self-compassion has been shown to reduce depression and anxiety and improve happiness and optimism (Neff, 2016). This idea is evoked vividly in the sensible recommendation in airline safety guidelines to put our own oxygen masks in place before helping others with theirs. Such advice is also regularly given to firefighters and other rescue service personal that the first person they must always ensure the safety of is themselves. Just like these people are of no use if they are hurt or in danger, if nurses do not practice regular self-care, they are less able to be present and caring for their patients. Often, however, nurses may forego their own self-care in the process of caring for others.

According to the ANA health risk appraisal, over two thirds (68%) of the nurses reported putting the health, safety, and wellness of their patients before their own. This means it is essential to educate both nurses and their employers on the importance of nurse self-care.

This appraisal also showed that 82% of nurses felt they were at risk of suffering significant workplace stress and half of all respondents had been bullied in some manner in the workplace. Yet nurses can only give the best care to patients when they are at their own best physically, mentally, and emotionally. There is, thus, a need for nurses to have ongoing resources to help maintain their resilience in the workplace and in life. Regular assessment of self-care practices is essential, and being able to feel connected with others at work and outside of work can help diffuse stress, build resilient networks, and refocus attention on what has meaning and purpose.

Often nurses may feel alone or worry that they will be judged by others for feeling overwhelmed and unable to cope with work stressors or difficult situations. It is crucial, therefore, that there is support to set aside time for a debriefing session, led by those trained in emotional first aid or nurse managers, with the goal to seek to understand what happened in an adverse event and prevent future harm. Linking nurses with peer support without delay could be the first step in processing their feelings and identifying additional resources to help them heal, such as an employee assistance program. Discussion and support should include having permission to take time away from work for a break that is needed for self-care.

### Preventative Strategies to Build Resilience

When events happen unexpectedly in the workplace there is a need for both in-the-moment response and after response to prevent the second victim's phenomenon. Equally as important is to move toward prevention and provide health promotion strategies that will enhance nurses' ability to bounce back quicker after these events and sustain resilience. Studies have investigated the relation of resilience to factors such as job satisfaction, emotional exhaustion, PTSD, and burnout (Manzano García, Calvo, & Carlos, 2012; Matos, Neushotz, Griffin, & Fitzpatrick, 2010; Mealer, Jones, & Moss, 2012). Based on the outcomes of this research, it is possible to say that positive social relationships, optimism, spirituality, and having a resilient role model all have a positive impact on nurses' resilience levels, while nurses with a low level of resilience experience more emotional exhaustion and job dissatisfaction.

There are several interventions that can be considered to build or improve resilience in nurses. These can be classed into three categories: (a) improving individual resiliency, (b) organizing the work environment, and (c) increasing support sources.

Interventions for improving individual resilience might include development and participation in stress management and resiliency programs, mindfulness programs and resources, mentorship and orientation programs, unit socialization programs, worksite wellness programs or relaxation training programs that guide staff with use of techniques like paced deep breathing, meditation, progressive muscle relaxation, or guided imagery.

In relation to the work environment, a systematic review commissioned by the UK's Department of Health reviewed a large number of international healthy workplace interventions and recommended system changes to improve healthcare staff's health and well-being (Brand et al., 2017). These include the identification of, and response to, local needs; engaging staff at all levels; and the involvement or support of leadership at all levels in healthcare.

Interventions that are associated with the work environment might also include development and support for structured and unstructured time for staff to gather and get support from one another or debrief. This would be an opportunity to reflect on the practice of others and provide support to each other. Another work environment intervention would include having leadership support for workplace well-being activities and education that might include short exercises, guided relaxation, guidance for self-care applications, and updates on the latest on evidence for health and well-being. Some medical facilities have taken steps to provide workplace behavioral response teams and/or employee assistance programs that offer structured debriefing and individual counseling for self-care when there is a significant event on a work unit.

The third category of interventions is to find ways to increase support sources for staff nurses. This can be accomplished through use of the specific work environment resources mentioned earlier but also by actively exploring individually and in the workplaces ways to improve positive and supportive relationships. This may be an important part of creating and supporting mentorship and orientation programs and may also include training on empathic communication skills to help us compassionately support each other and the patients we serve.

While stress reduction techniques may be helpful for individuals in the short-term, a long-term plan for success in this area will rely upon organizational responses to the sources of added stress, and support for preventing stress in the first place (Press Ganey, 2018). The Press Ganey (2018) report indicates this can be accomplished in a number of ways. These are: improving the function of healthcare teams; systematically identifying work that does not add value, or that can be streamlined to prevent unnecessary work; communicating to employees the ultimate goal of healthcare provider's work, which is to meet patients' needs and reduce suffering; creating an environment where employees are able to support one another; and, placing emphasis on the support of the values and culture of the organization.

## CONCLUSION

Secondary trauma, burnout, and intention to leave the profession are major concerns that arise as a result of nurses failing to adequately deal with stress caused by such stressors as overwork, bullying, and violence in the workplace. Healthcare professionals throughout the developed world report higher levels of sickness, absence, dissatisfaction, distress, and burnout at work than staff in other sectors. Common stressors are work overload; role conflicts; experiences of aggression; lack of time; staffing issues; shift work; lack of self-care; poor job-related interpersonal relationships; feeling powerless to provide quality care; struggling with competing demands; ensuring excellent patient care; uncertainty concerning treatment; death and dying; conflict with doctors, peers, and supervisors; and inadequate emotional preparation, just to name a few. Nurses are now dealing with an increase in violent behavior in the workplace and recognition of the second victim's phenomenon. There is a growing call to go beyond the triple aim of healthcare delivery that includes improving patient experience and outcomes and reducing costs, to include a fourth aim: improving healthcare staff's experience of healthcare delivery.

## LEARNING ACTIVITIES

1. Think about a stressful situation when you dealt with a patient with a mental health situation. How did you handle it in-the-moment and after the event, and what would you do differently in the future?

2. What specific actions did Kristin employ in her situation to mitigate stress and to contribute to a safe patient outcome?
3. Can you identify how Kristin used empathic communication techniques in her interactions with her patient? What did she convey in her communication to the patient, and how may have that impacted the patient's response?
4. Sample activities you can try for preventive, in-the-moment, and ongoing stress management:
   - Identify people who can support you at work and in your home life that will listen to you with the intention of listening without judgment or an attempt to solve the problem.
   - Identify self-care activities you can do daily, for example: deep breathing, mindful walk, focused attention, meditation or imagery, affirmations, break time to rest, refresh and replenish.
   - Reflect on resources available in your clinical facility/community that could be utilized to mitigate nurse stress.
   - Create a mindfulness station in your work setting or home environment—what would they include?

## Acknowledgment

The authors wish to acknowledge the contributions of Dr. Amit Sood, Professor of Medicine at the Mayo Clinic.

## REFERENCES

Allen, R. C., & Palk, G. (2018). Development of recommendations and guidelines for strengthening resilience in emergency department nurses. *Traumatology*, 24, 148–156. doi:10.1037/trm0000141

American Nurses Association. (2018). Healthy Nurse Healthy Nation Grand Challenge. Retrieved from http://www.healthynursehealthynation.org/en

Brand, S. L., Coon, J. T., Fleming, L. E., Carroll, L., Bethel, A., & Wyatt, K. (2017). Whole-system approaches to improving the health and wellbeing of healthcare workers: A systematic review. *PloS One*, 12(12), e0188418. doi:10.1371/journal.pone.0188418

Brandford, A. A., & Reed, D. B. (2016). Depression in registered nurses: A state of the science. *Workplace Health & Safety*, 64(10), 488–511. doi:10.1177/2165079916653415

Centers for Disease Control and Prevention. (2015). Occupational traumatic injuries among workers in health care facilities—United States, 2012–2014. *Morbidity and Mortality Weekly Report*, 64(15), 405–410.

Choi, S. H., & Lee, H. (2017). Workplace violence against nurses in Korea and its impact on professional quality of life and turnover intention. *Journal of Nursing Management, 25*(7), 508–518. doi:10.1111/jonm.12488

Duncan, S. M., Hyndamn, K., Estabrooks, C. A., Hesketh, K., Humphrey, C. K., Wong, J. S., ... Giovannetti, P. (2016). Nurses' experience of violence in Alberta and British Columbia hospitals. *Canadian Journal of Nursing Research Archive, 32*(4). Retrieved from http://cjnr.archive.mcgill.ca/issue/view/174

Gates, D. M., Gillespie, G. L., & Succop, P. (2011). Violence against nurses and its impact on stress and productivity. *Nursing Economics, 29*(2), 59.

Grawitch, M. J., Gottschalk, M., & Munz, D. C. (2006). The path to a healthy workplace: A critical review linking healthy workplace practices, employee well-being, and organizational improvements. *Consulting Psychology Journal: Practice and Research, 58*(3), 129. doi:10.1037/1065-9293.58.3.129

Happell, B., Reid-Searl, K., Dwyer, T., Caperchione, C. M., Gaskin, C. J., & Burke, K. J. (2013). How nurses cope with occupational stress outside their workplaces. *Collegian, 20*(3), 195–199. doi:10.1016/j.colegn.2012.08.003

Kyeong, S., Kim, J., Kim, D. J., Kim, H. E., & Kim, J. J. (2017). Effects of gratitude meditation on neural network functional connectivity and brain-heart coupling. *Scientific Reports, 7*(1), 5058. doi:10.1038/s41598-017-05520-9

Manzano García, G., Calvo, A., & Carlos, J. (2012). Emotional exhaustion of nursing staff: Influence of emotional annoyance and resilience. *International Nursing Review, 59*(1), 101–107. doi:10.1111/j.1466-7657.2011.00927.x

Matos, P. S., Neushotz, L. A., Griffin, M. T. Q., & Fitzpatrick, J. J. (2010). An exploratory study of resilience and job satisfaction among psychiatric nurses working in inpatient units. *International Journal of Mental Health Nursing, 19*(5), 307–312. doi:10.1111/j.1447-0349.2010.00690.x

Mealer, M., Jones, J., & Moss, M. (2012). A qualitative study of resilience and post-traumatic stress disorder in United States ICU nurses. *Intensive Care Medicine, 38*(9), 1445–1451. doi:10.1007/s00134-012-2600-6

Mills, J., Wand, T., & Fraser, J. (2015). On self-compassion and self-care in nursing: Selfish or essential for compassionate care? *International Journal of Nursing Studies, 52*(4), 791–793. doi:10.1016/j.ijnurstu.2014.10.009

Neff, K. D. (2016). Self-compassion. In I. Ivtzan & T. Lomas (Eds.), *Mindfulness in positive psychology: The science of meditation and wellbeing* (pp. 37–50). London, UK: Routledge.

Neumann, M., Bensing, J., Mercer, S., Ernstmann, N., Ommen, O., & Pfaff, H. (2009). Analyzing the "nature" and "specific effectiveness" of clinical empathy: A theoretical overview and contribution towards a theory-based research agenda. *Patient Education and Counseling, 74*(3), 339–346. doi:10.1016/j.pec.2008.11.013

Pekurinen, V., Willman, L., Virtanen, M., Kivimäki, M., Vahtera, J., & Välimäki, M. (2017). Patient aggression and the wellbeing of nurses: A cross-sectional survey study in psychiatric and non-psychiatric settings. *International Journal of Environmental Research and Public Health, 14*(10), 1245. doi:10.3390/ijerph14101245

Pines, A. M. (2017). Burnout: An existential perspective. In W. Schaufeli, C. Maslach, & T. Marek (Eds.), *Professional burnout* (pp. 33–51). London, UK: Routledge.

Press Ganey. (2018). White paper burnout and resilience: A framework for data analysis and a positive path forward. South Bend, IN. Retrieved from http://images.healthcare.pressganey.com/Web/PressGaneyAssociatesInc/%7B8 40f3614-c459-4dd5-8786-b4915eddc06c%7D_2018_PG_Burnout_Resilience.pdf

Price, S. L. (2009). Becoming a nurse: A meta-study of early professional socialization and career choice in nursing. *Journal of Advanced Nursing, 65*(1), 11–19. doi:10.1111/j.1365-2648.2008.04839.x

Quillivan, R. R., Burlison, J. D., Browne, E. K., Scott, S. D., & Hoffman, J. M. (2016). Patient safety culture and the second victim phenomenon: Connecting culture to staff distress in nurses. *Joint Commission Journal on Quality and Patient Safety, 42*(8), AP1–AP2. doi:10.1016/S1553-7250(16)42053-2

Romppanen, J., & Häggman-Laitila, A. (2017). Interventions for nurses' well-being at work: A quantitative systematic review. *Journal of Advanced Nursing, 73*(7), 1555–1569. doi:10.1111/jan.13210

Scott, S., Hirschinger, L., Cox, K., McCoig, M., Hahn-Cover, K., Epperly, K., . . . Hall, L. (2010). Caring for our own: Deploying a systemwide second victim rapid response team. *The Joint Commission Journal on Quality and Patient Safety, 36*(5), 233–240. doi:10.1016/S1553-7250(10)36038-7

Seys, D., Wu, A. W., Gerven, E. V., Vleugels, A., Euwema, M., Panella, M., . . . Vanhaecht, K. (2013). Health care professionals as second victims after adverse events: A systematic review. *Evaluation & The Health Professions, 36*(2), 135–162. doi:10.1177/0163278712458918

Silverman, J., Kurtz, S., & Draper, J. (1998). *Teaching and Learning Communication Skills in Medicine*. London, UK: Radcliffe Medical Press Ltd.

Sood, A. (2010). *Train your brain engage your heart transform your life: A two-step program to enhance attention; decrease stress; cultivate peace, joy and resilience; and practice presence with love: A course in Attention & Interpretation Therapy*. Rochester, MN: Morning Dew Publications.

Sood, A. (2013). *The Mayo Clinic guide to stress-free living*. Philadelphia, PA: Da Capo Press.

Speroni, K. G., Fitch, T., Dawson, E., Dugan, L., & Atherton, M. (2014). Incidence and cost of nurse workplace violence perpetrated by hospital patients or patient visitors. *Journal of Emergency Nursing, 40*(3), 218–228. doi:10.1016/j.jen.2013.05.014

Suchman, A. L., Markakis, K., Beckman, H. B., & Frankel, R. (1997). A model of empathic communication in the medical interview. *Journal of the American Medical Association, 277*(8), 678–682. doi:10.1001/jama.1997.03540320082047

Van Gerven, E., Bruyneel, L., Panella, M., Euwema, M., Sermeus, W., & Vanhaecht, K. (2016). Psychological impact and recovery after involvement in a patient safety incident: A repeated measures analysis. *British Medical Journal Open, 6*(8), e011403. doi:10.1136/bmjopen-2016-011403

# 10

# Fostering Resilience in Others

Sandra Sharp

## INTRODUCTION

People are often asked "If you could have dinner with any great leader from history, or even a current inspirational leader, who would it be?" Nominees might include Abraham Lincoln who enacted measures, despite vehement opposition, to abolish slavery; Mahatma Gandhi who led thousands of oppressed Indians to conduct peaceful protests against British Imperialism and gain independence; or Martin Luther King Jr. who motivated people across the world to believe in a world of equality and energized the Civil Rights Movement. Nurses or nursing students might well invite guests such as Florence Nightingale, persistent advocate for nursing's professionalization; or Australian nurse Vivian Bullwinkel who, in the Second World War, managed to survive a massacre that killed many of her fellow nurses by hiding her wounds, and then surviving on a deserted island, before surrendering to the enemy and becoming a leader in a women's prison camp (McAllister, 2014).

During that dinner party, guests might ask these great leaders for advice about how to lead others effectively, and how to relate to others in ways that are meaningful, effective, and visionary. Perhaps they would like to know how to make a positive and lasting impact as a leader. It is likely that in asking this, guests are particularly interested in the resilience of these leaders, in the factors that kept them going even in the face of intense opposition or personal suffering. I have a hunch that each of them would, in their own way, agree that resilience involves being true to yourself rather than trying to be someone you think others expect or want you to be (Smith-Trudeau, 2015). At first glance, this advice might seem a little vague but it points to authenticity, teamwork, perseverance in the face of opposition, consistency between words and actions, and ultimately being easy to follow. These are all important aspects of resilient leadership that each of these great leaders exemplified.

*Many great leaders demonstrate authenticity, teamwork, persistence, and integrity—vital resilience strategies.*

## AUTHENTICITY AND VISION

Authentic leaders act in ways that are congruent with their values, beliefs and convictions. Sometimes this action occurs despite great personal cost. Consider, for instance, Nelson Mandela the anti-Apartheid activist who spent 27 years in prison, separated from his family, before his eventual release and subsequent Presidency of South Africa. In the entire period of his imprisonment, his commitment to fight Apartheid did not waver. Mandela led with purpose, values, and integrity, and was "the author of his own story" (Avolio & Gardner, 2005). That is, he had a vision of a new reality in South Africa, in which Black and White people were equal, and he lived his life according to that vision.

In common with other authentic leaders (such as Gandhi, Bullwinkel, and King), Mandela also displayed characteristics such as empathy, integrity, and warmth that made him relatable and trustworthy (Waite, McKinney, Smith-Glasgow, & Meloy, 2014). Such characteristics make such leaders easy to follow. Furthermore, Mandela demonstrated that authenticity is not about following a "party-line" or conforming to organizational expectations. Instead, he chose to act according to his own values and, moreover, he did this at great personal cost (Murphy, Duggan, & Joseph, 2013). Just imagine how different history might be if Mandela had conformed to the status quo and remained silent. Equally, nurse leaders need authenticity and vision to ensure their team remains unified and given clear direction and a firm value base.

## A TEAM WITH CONFLICTING VISION AND VALUES

Recently, I conducted an ethnography of nursing teamwork in a busy surgical ward and found numerous obstacles to unity, direction, and value-based practice (Sharp, McAllister, & Broadbent, 2017). On each shift, there were seven registered nurses, one appointed as team leader for that shift, a clinical educator, and charge nurse to care for 30 patients. (Names are changed in the following.) The day began with handover before the pace increased in earnest with medication rounds, patients to prepare for surgery, and postoperative patients to monitor, as well as infusions, epidurals, and wounds to manage. There were also drains to remove, home discharges to organize, medical rounds to attend, personal hygiene care to deliver, phone calls to field, and emergent events to respond to. On top of all this, nurses were under immense pressure to meet a series of new organizational targets required by the recently introduced National Quality and Health Service Standards (Australia) and felt overwhelmed by the new paperwork designed to show that all these targets were being met.

There seemed to be a tacit understanding within the team that each individual nurse would ensure that all tasks were completed before handing over to the next shift. Beth had recently joined the team and described how she quite quickly got the message that efficiency was highly valued, that leaving work for nurses on the next shift to complete was unacceptable, and that—given these priorities—person-centered care was not the highest priority.

An incident occurred one morning while Beth was receiving handover at the bedside. Bedside handover was a new strategy formally introduced by Shelly, the nurse in charge, who was attempting to operationalize the hospital policy of "shared decision-making"—a way to encourage patients to be actively involved in their own care planning, and for nurses to be collaborative and respectful of patients in their reporting (Cegala, 2011). Beth and her colleagues for the shift were listening to a report from the night duty staff about John, a patient who had a below the knee amputation and an epidural in situ. June, the patient's daughter, interrupted discussions to request that her father be given his medication. She explained, apologetically, to the team that John needed to take his phosphate binders before breakfast because he had renal disease, was on dialysis, and that this drug needed to be consumed with food to facilitate the absorption and excretion of phosphate. Beth was just about to reassure June that they would be dispensed immediately. Before she had a chance to speak, however, Irene, a nurse of similar rank to Beth, but more experienced, said dismissively, "We'll get to that in a minute." She shot Beth a look that implied this was the last word on the matter and Beth kept silent. The team moved to the next patient's bedside and, by this time, the breakfasts had arrived. June, quite bravely, interrupted again. This time she crisply asked, "Can we have them now please?" Despite this request, Irene responded in an exasperated tone. "Look, these girls have been going all night and need to get home, we'll be with your Dad shortly!" There was an uncomfortable silence, but no one dared move to get John's medication.

Later, Irene highlighted to me, as the researcher, the importance of keeping up with the workload and not adding to anyone's work burdens. "We just have to keep focused, otherwise we'll drown," she said. She went on to describe how she felt successful and valued by others in the team when she left the ward having worked hard to achieve everything she had set out to do. Feeling a part of the team was an aspect of her work that she particularly valued and she saw it as her role to ensure others complied with expectations and did their fair share.

The conflict in this situation was located in a clash between personal and team values. Beth had a deep desire to provide person-centered care and really supported Shelley's improvement strategies, but the team was driven by a need to complete tasks swiftly in order to meet deadlines and prevent overload. Over time, Beth learned that team priorities were paramount because she experienced some passive-aggressive responses when handing over tasks she had not been able to complete, and often felt the ire of colleagues like Irene. Beth also frequently felt excluded from the team and unfulfilled as a nurse.

## LESSONS LEARNED FROM THE STORY

In this situation it was the informal team leader, Irene, who exerted significant cultural power over the group of nurses in the ward. Similarly, Harrowing and Mill (2010) explain that informal leaders have covert ways of directing and controlling the actions of others. Informal leaders tend to use the promise of acceptance and belonging, and implicitly the threat of social exclusion, to encourage workers to comply with cultural rules above personal values. In the scenario described, people conformed to the team expectations just to gain acceptance rather than acting according to their own values and standards. Beth exemplified this in suppressing her own values and, instead, complying with Irene's expectations. However, compliance can be detrimental to a nurse's well-being and resilience. It is known that nurses who do not act in ways that are congruent with their values are more likely to experience moral distress and burnout (Oh & Gastmans, 2015). Therefore, although being in the team can facilitate belonging and social support, when the team is under pressure it can also be detrimental to authenticity.

### Maintaining Resilience in a Dynamic Healthcare Environment

The healthcare environments in busy clinical settings in the UK, United States, and Australia are characterized as typical bureaucracies. They function with hierarchies, written rules, and specialized division of labor. They value efficiency over satisfaction, and the environment tends toward the impersonal (Bridges et al., 2013). Healthcare is an expensive business, and thus decisions that involve cost- and time-saving will be favored over the more complex and hard to solve problems of patient anxiety, frustration, and anger, or staff shortages, moral distress, and feelings of powerlessness (Varcoe, Pauly, Storch, Newton, & Makaroff, 2012). Nursing work is increasingly being measured, quantified, and critiqued, placing nurses under rising pressure to perform efficiently (Sharp et al., 2017). In such an impersonal, managerial environment, nurses might perceive that they have very little autonomy over how their values are supported and their work is planned. This, coupled with increasing patient acuity, and increasing technological demands, creates a very stressful work environment for many nurses (Brady Germain & Cummings, 2010). As a consequence, compassion fatigue, burnout, and the intention to leave are prevalent. These are major reasons why leaders need to step up to unify and support teams and, thus, promote employee resilience (Trybou et al., 2014).

> *Compassion fatigue is prevalent in health bureaucracies—a major reason why leaders need to step up to unify and support teams.*

## LEADERSHIP UNDER PRESSURE

It is clear that in pressured environments such as the contemporary healthcare system, leaders are necessary to help motivate teams, to validate their adherence to values even when resources are tight, and to lighten the atmosphere so that negative emotions dissipate and a sense of shared purpose is renewed. A memorable example of leadership under pressure is the story of the British polar explorer, Ernest Shackleton. A summary of his story is told here, and then reflected upon in order to identify leadership skills and examples of resilience.

At the turn of the 20th century, Shackleton had a dream to become the first person to set foot on the South Pole. Unfortunately for him, Roald Edmundson reached the pole first. However, Shackleton did not despair or give up his dream; rather, he set himself a new goal of crossing the Antarctic (Shackleton, 2002). He gathered together a team of shipmates, raised considerable funds to support the venture, and even arranged a second ship to lay a supply of food and fuel along the route. With preparations complete, the crew set sail just a few days after the outbreak of the First World War. Half way through the trans-Atlantic crossing, the ship, aptly named the *Endurance*, encountered blizzard conditions and eventually became trapped in ice. The group faced a horrible dilemma—stay in the ship and hope for rescue or move to shore and try to survive. Shackleton convinced the crew to abandon ship in a region that had not before been explored because, he reasoned, they could not be victims of inaction. The group agreed but found that they had no means of communication to send out a rescue signal.

Shackleton organized the crew into teams to set up camp on the ice. Shackleton made it his business to get to know each of the crewmen and nurtured and developed their capabilities. He knew that inactivity, cold, and lack of purpose could have a devastating impact on the crew's morale, so he ensured that the men were busy and that their skills and abilities were put to good use. The scientists in the group were encouraged to collect and catalog specimens and the ship's carpenter was tasked to make improvements to a small open boat that Shackleton would later use to summon help.

At one point, the unity of the team came under threat. Six months of hardship in the freezing cold and no likelihood of rescue had led to one person criticizing the captain's leadership. Shackleton became aware of this potential mutiny. Immediately, the man was confronted and reminded of his legal and professional duties. Shackleton also subscribed to the motto "keep your friends close and your enemies closer" and located any potential dissenters in the tent next to his. Eventually, Shackleton realized that rescue was unlikely, and he made the decision to risk a thousand-mile journey by boat to a whaling station, where he knew help would be available. He chose a small group of five men to make the journey with him including a skilled navigator, two strong sailors, and the dissenter who had almost caused a mutiny. Despite the man's potential treachery, Shackleton knew his skills as a carpenter would be vital to keep the boat seaworthy.

In his absence, Shackleton's second in command was promoted to the rank of captain. He knew that routine was important and each day got the men to pack up their belongings in anticipation of rescue. They lived there for 2 years before being rescued, maintaining the daily routines of hunting, photographing, collecting, cataloguing, and socializing. Astonishingly, not a single crew member died during this time. The remarkable survival of the entire crew was attributed to Shackleton's leadership skills, which inspired confidence, collective action, perseverance, and optimism in his crew (Harland, Harrison, Jones, & Reiter-Palmon, 2004).

## APPLYING THE LESSONS TO LEADERSHIP OF TEAMS IN NURSING

According to some researchers (Harland et al., 2004), Shackleton prioritized the welfare and well-being of his men. His devotion to them then became reciprocal. Team cohesion was also highly valued. Not only did Shackleton provide firm leadership, he expected his followers to play their part and even to step into leadership should his abilities be compromised. The crew of the *Endurance* was a united team; faced with the same adversities and a shared goal, they banded together to pool their strengths and resources. They refused the possibilities of division, personal egos, and competition. On his part, Shackleton nurtured and developed his men, enabling each to achieve his best. His optimism and self-belief became *their* optimism and self-belief. In these ways, the group proved to be resilient and ultimately survived. When leaders make it clear to teams that they share the same goals, unity of purpose can be achieved. Nurses, similarly, have shared goals—the delivery of high-quality patient care and workplace satisfaction (McCormack & McCance, 2006).

> *When leaders make it clear to teams that they share the same goals, unity of purpose can be achieved.*

Shackleton was an admired mentor. He wanted to see his team survive, and he wanted each of them to gain skills, and to show courage and persistence. His faith in his team members enhanced each individual's self-belief and resilience. Studies in nursing have also shown that when nurses are coached and mentored they are better equipped to perform their role and they enjoy their work because they feel supported and hold a sense of group belonging (Faithfull-Byrne et al., 2017).

Shackleton modeled persistence, adaptability, resilience, and optimism and put his concern for his men into action. On one occasion, he gave up his own mittens, suffering frostbite as a consequence, so that the photographer in his team could continue to record their epic journey. He earned the respect of his men because he too experienced their hardships and was fully engaged in the work of survival. In nursing, leaders who model the possibility of staying true to values while also aspiring to technical competence are likely to earn respect and their behaviors will be imitated (Waite et al., 2014). By placing a high value on people, and acknowledging the challenges of tight resources and other pressures, leaders model perseverance in the face of complexity (Brady Germain & Cummings, 2010). This demands emotional intelligence and a manner of thinking about the situation that can be described as a systems way of thinking.

Emotional intelligence is defined as the ability to perceive, understand, process, and manage emotions (Karimi, Leggat, Donohue, Farrell, & Couper, 2014). Leaders who are emotionally intelligent report improved workplace performance and greater workplace satisfaction in themselves and in followers (Codier, Muneno, Franey, & Matsuura, 2010). Having a systems way of thinking is also exercising structural competence (Metzl & Hansen, 2014). In nursing, this is the awareness that the difficulties encountered at the ward level may be exacerbated by wider social issues such as those at the higher hospital policy level or within the health department more widely and, thus, as a leader it may be important to lobby and raise awareness of ward-based needs and inequalities at the policy level.

*Systems thinking involves seeing the interrelationships between smaller systems, such as how different systems in the human body interact, as well as how larger systems such as ward teams and hospital bureaucracies can affect each other.*

Nurses who are led by such leaders feel supported in the workplace and have greater optimism that change is possible (Delmatoff & Lazarus, 2014). Leaders who are striving for change are aware that self-containment and self-regulation are important in maintaining morale and the commitment within the team to maintain their persistence because change takes some time (Waite et al., 2014).

In the next story, each of the characters has their ability to cope and stay strong in the face of adversity seriously threatened.

## A STORY OF RECIPROCAL SUPPORT AND ENDURANCE

Jenny, a young woman newly diagnosed with cancer, relayed an encounter with a nurse that facilitated her movement from avoidance to acceptance. Jenny had come into the day center for her first chemotherapy treatment and despite the fact that she looked happy and engaged, she had spent the previous few days in a state of despair. Jenny's marriage had recently broken down after an experience of domestic violence, and she found herself a newly single parent with two pre-school children to care for. She feared for the future, wondering who would take care of her children.

Barbara was dreading work that day. On her last shift, a patient that she had become particularly fond of had died. Barbara was also concerned that hospital cutbacks were negatively impacting the service the staff could provide. There were fewer staff and she often felt rushed at work and unable to give patients the time she would have liked to provide them.

Barbara had never met Jenny before and was busily preparing the IV line to deliver her chemotherapy. Listening to Jenny's light chatter, and perhaps to what Jenny was not saying, Barbara leaned in, placed her hand on Jenny's, and said kindly, "It's okay. You can do this." In that moment, Jenny said she was stopped in her tracks. She described how this simple act was felt profoundly. Jenny said that Barbara's touch and hopeful words had touched her soul.

It was in that moment that Jenny began to acknowledge her fears and face them. It was also in that moment that Jenny felt empowered. She had the strength to triumph over her circumstance. Jenny described how she believed in Barbara's reassurance. Not only did the gentle words of encouragement touch Jenny emotionally and spiritually, they provided a foundation for building genuine resilience. When Jenny perceived that her nurse (and leader) believed in her ability to endure this health crisis, she too increased her resolve to remain strong no matter what might happen. Clearly the opinion of the leader matters to people and engenders confidence and self-belief. Equally, Barbara's self-belief was restored and she felt renewed, invigorated, and able to pursue her work once more grounded in her professional values.

### Learning From Jenny's Story

At the beginning of this story Jenny was displaying what has been described as avoidant coping (Harland et al., 2004). She was engaging in a flow of light chatter in an effort to forget the source of her stress. While this may appear outwardly similar to resilience, avoidant coping does not lead to the adaptation, personal growth, and development that are characteristic of resilience (Masten, 2001). Barbara perceived an inconsistency between the seriousness of having a first dose of chemotherapy and her intuitive sense of anxiety in the patient and

Jenny's stream of light chatter. Barbara had the courage to act with authenticity, by communicating concern as well as optimism and this facilitated Jenny's self-reflection and forward movement.

Masten (2001) argues that in order for a person to be declared resilient, that person must have first faced adversity and triumphed. Harland et al. (2004) agree and add that resilience can only be developed when a threat is encountered and faced, leading to adaptation and personal growth. Masten (2001) further contends that if an individual has not experienced a threat, their resilience has not yet been tested and therefore not proven. For Masten, resilience is not an extraordinary power that only special people have, but is, instead, a common human adaptive process facilitated by negotiating and resolving risks. As has been explored previously in this volume, the combination of personal factors such as a positive self-concept together with social factors such as positive role models and supportive relationships are known to promote resilience.

In Jenny's story we reveal that Barbara's caring actions were a catalyst for resilience for both patient and nurse. It has been recognized that the therapeutic potential of a nurse–patient relationship can only be realized once a genuine connection is made (Perraud et al., 2006). Touch and gentle words helped Barbara make this connection, and this therapeutic relationship benefited both she and Jenny. From Jenny's perspective, the individualized compassion helped her move from a problem focus and denial to a solution-focused frame of mind. From Barbara's perspective, she felt grounded and renewed because she was providing care congruent with her professional and personal values.

In acting to promote Jenny's resilience, Barbara promoted her own. Nursing is a profession characterized by the constant giving of self and is associated with a high degree of emotional labor or effort. It involves regulating one's own emotions so that patients feel safe and cared for (Bartram, Casimir, Djurkovic, Leggat, & Stanton, 2012). Working in an oncology unit, Barbara was constantly faced with suffering and it would have been emotionally draining work. Without her own resilience, she would experience compassion fatigue and burnout (McAllister, 2013). The temptation can be to revert to task-focused, impersonal care, just to survive emotionally. However, resilience enabled Barbara to deliver care according to her professional values and philosophy. This is because resilience intersects with tacit knowledge needed not only to survive, but thrive in nursing (McDonald, Jackson, Wilkes, & Vickers, 2012). Furthermore, the ability to deliver care that is congruent with personal values is positively associated with workplace satisfaction, and it is known that workplace satisfaction is a mediator of workplace stress and a further promoter of resilience (Lehuluante, Nilsson, & Edvardsson, 2012). Thus, a cycle ensues that is mutually beneficial to all members of the team.

Throughout this story, Barbara displayed many of the characteristics of effective leadership. By connecting with Jenny, she was authentic and demonstrated an optimism that became reciprocal. She inspired a shared vision that Jenny could triumph; she strengthened Jenny and ultimately valued and encouraged her. Aspiring leaders would do well to follow her example, no matter how large or small the team they are leading.

## CONCLUSION

Resilience is not only necessary for professional job satisfaction in nursing, it is vital for personal good health and well-being. This chapter outlined some of the challenges of stepping up to leadership in the very challenging environment of contemporary healthcare. Leadership is required at all levels from the nurse–patient relationship to leading teams under pressure. Leaders need to be resilient and they need to promote resilience in others. A key quality that might facilitate resilience in leadership is that of authenticity, the ability to stay true to the values that are held. Ultimately, effective leaders must promote the well-being and development needs of their followers so that they too can be resilient and rise to the challenge of leadership.

### LEARNING ACTIVITIES

1. Outline how you would approach the leadership role within the team depicted in the story about teams under pressure. What potential challenges and opportunities might you experience? What are your strategies for building personal and team resilience?

In answering this essay question you might consider:

- The concept of resilience
- Knowing yourself and your values, your leadership style and personal impact
- Strategies for effective communication and relationship building
- Engendering a shared vision and keeping the vision foremost
- Change-management strategies
- Challenges might include resistance to change, suspicion of newcomers and new ideas, people being set in their ways, resource implications and shortages
- Opportunities might include a fresh vision, professional and personal development in self and followers, untapped skills and abilities

2. Utilizing an example from your clinical practice, critically evaluate a leadership approach that facilitated resilience or perhaps missed an opportunity to do so.

In answering this question you might consider:

- The concept of resilience and challenges to resilience
- A situation where you needed to implement a change or quality improvement or lead a new team
- Leadership styles and their effectiveness in different situations

# REFERENCES

Avolio, B., J., & Gardner, W., L. (2005). Authentic Leadership development: Getting to the root of positive forms of leadership. *The Leadership Quarterly, 16*(2005), 315–338. doi:10.1016/j.leaqua.2005.03.001

Bartram, T., Casimir, G., Djurkovic, N., Leggat, S. G., & Stanton, P. (2012). Do perceived high performance work systems influence the relationship between emotional labour, burnout and intention to leave? A study of Australian nurses. *Journal of Advanced Nursing, 68*(7), 1567–1578. doi:10.1111/j.1365-2648.2012.05968.x

Brady Germain, P., & Cummings, G. G. (2010). The influence of nursing leadership on nurse performance: A systematic literature review. *Journal of Nursing Management, 18*(4), 425–439. doi:10.1111/j.1365-2834.2010.01100.x

Bridges, J., Nicholson, C., Maben, J., Pope, C., Flatley, M., Wilkinson, C., . . . Tziggili, M. (2013). Capacity for care: Meta-ethnography of acute care nurses' experiences of the nurse–patient relationship. *Journal of Advanced Nursing, 69*(4), 760–772.

Cegala, D. (2011). An exploration of factors promoting patient participation in primary care medical interviews. *Health Communication, 26*(5), 427–436. doi:10.1080/10410236.2011.552482

Codier, E., Muneno, L., Franey, K., & Matsuura, F. (2010). Is emotional intelligence an important concept for nursing practice? *Journal of Psychiatric & Mental Health Nursing, 17*(10), 940–948. doi:10.1111/j.1365-2850.2010.01610.x

Delmatoff, J., & Lazarus, I. R. (2014). The most effective leadership style for the new landscape of healthcare. *Journal of Healthcare Management, 59*(4), 245–249. doi:10.1097/00115514-201407000-00003

Faithfull-Byrne, A., Thompson, L., Schafer, K. W., Elks, M., Jaspers, J., Welch, A., . . . Moss, C. (2017). Clinical coaches in nursing and midwifery practice: Facilitating point of care workplace learning and development. *Collegian, 24*(4), 403–410. doi:10.1016/j.colegn.2016.06.001

Harland, L., Harrison, W., Jones, J., & Reiter-Palmon, R. (2004). Leadership behaviors and subordinate resilience. *Journal of Leadership & Organizational Studies, 11*(2), 2–14. doi:10.1177/107179190501100202

Harrowing, J. N., & Mill, J. (2010). Moral distress among Ugandan nurses providing HIV care: A critical ethnography. *International Journal of Nursing Studies, 47*, 723–731. doi:10.1016/j.ijnurstu.2009.11.010

Karimi, L., Leggat, S. G., Donohue, L., Farrell, G., & Couper, G. E. (2014). Emotional rescue: The role of emotional intelligence and emotional labour on well-being and job-stress among community nurses. *Journal of Advanced Nursing, 70*(1), 176–186. doi:10.1111/jan.12185

Lehuluante, A., Nilsson, A., & Edvardsson, D. (2012). The influence of a person-centred psychosocial unit climate on satisfaction with care and work. *Journal of Nursing Management, 20*(3), 319–325. doi:10.1111/j.1365-2834.2011.01286.x

Masten, A. (2001). Ordinary magic: Resilience processes in development. *American Psychologist, 56*(3), 11. doi:10.1037/0003-066X.56.3.227

McAllister, M. (2013). Resilience: A personal attribute, social process and key professional resource for the enhancement of the nursing role. *Professioni Infermieristiche, 66*(1), 55–62. doi:10.7429/pi.2013.661055

McAllister, M. (2014). Vivian Bullwinkel: A model of resilience and a symbol of strength. *Collegian, 22*, 135–141. doi:10.1016/j.colegn.2013.12.006

McCormack, B., & McCance, T. V. (2006). Development of a framework for person-centred nursing. *Journal of Advanced Nursing, 56*(5), 472–479. doi:10.1111/j.1365-2648.2006.04042.x

McDonald, G., Jackson, D., Wilkes, L., & Vickers, M. (2012). A work-based educational intervention to support the development of personal resilience in nurses and midwives. *Nurse Education Today, 32*, 6. doi:10.1016/j.nedt.2011.04.012

Metzl, J. M., & Hansen, H., (2014). Structural competency: Theorizing a new medical engagement with stigma and inequality. *Social Science & Medicine, 103*, 126–133. doi:10.1016/j.socscimed.2013.06.032

Murphy, D., Duggan, M., & Joseph, S. (2013). Relationship-based social work and its compatibility with the person-centred approach: Principled versus instrumental perspectives. *British Journal of Social Work, 43*(4), 703–719. doi:10.1093/bjsw/bcs003

Oh, Y., & Gastmans, C. (2015). Moral distress experienced by nurses: A quantitative literature review. *Nursing Ethics, 22*(1), 15–31. doi:10.1177/0969733013502803

Perraud, S., Delaney, K. R., Carlson-Sabelli, L., Johnson, M. E., Shephard, R., & Paun, O. (2006). Advanced practice psychiatric mental health nursing, finding our core: The therapeutic relationship in 21st century. *Perspectives in Psychiatric Care, 42*(4), 215–226. doi:10.1111/j.1744-6163.2006.00097.x

Shackleton, A. (2002). Tending Sir Ernest's legacy: An interview with Alexandra Shackleton (Ernest Shackleton's granddaughter). Retrieved from http://www.pbs .org/wgbh/nova/shackleton/1914/alexandra.html

Sharp, S., McAllister, M., & Broadbent, M. (2017). The tension between person centred and task focused care in an acute surgical setting: A critical ethnography. *Collegian, 25*, 6.

Smith-Trudeau, P. (2015). The journey to authentic nursing leadership at the point of care. *Vermont Nurse Connection, 18*(4), 3. Retrieved from https://www.nursingald.com/ articles/14097-the-journey-to-authentic-nursing-leadership-at-the-point-of-care

Trybou, J., Germonpre, S., Janssens, H., Casini, A., Braeckman, L., Bacquer, D. D., & Clays, E. (2014). Job-related stress and sickness absence among Belgian nurses: A prospective study. *Journal of Nursing Scholarship, 46*(4), 292. doi:10.1111/jnu.12075

Varcoe, C., Pauly, B., Storch, J., Newton, L., & Makaroff, K. (2012). Nurses' perceptions of and responses to morally distressing situations. *Nursing Ethics, 19*(4), 488–500. doi:10.1177/0969733011436025

Waite, R., McKinney, N., Smith-Glasgow, M. E., & Meloy, F. A. (2014). The embodiment of authentic leadership. *Journal of Professional Nursing, 30*(4), 282–291. doi:10.1016/j.profnurs.2013.11.004

# 11

# Maintaining Your Resilience

Jane Brannan, Mary de Chesnay, Patricia L. Hart, and Margaret McAllister

## INTRODUCTION

The purpose of this chapter is to provide various ideas for relaxing and letting go of the tension from work. Although these strategies may be familiar, when nurses are actively experiencing stress from high-pressure jobs—as a new graduate trying to acculturate to the new practice setting, for example—they may forget to implement them. Ruminating about what happened that day at work and taking shortcuts such as eating fast food and watching television, instead of a healthy meal and exercising, is all too easy. However, nurses must remember that work is only *one* aspect of life, all-consuming although that work may seem at times. To be a success in nursing, a nurse must be a success in life. The ideas in this chapter will help nurses to remember that life is much more than work. Taking time for some of the suggested activities, or others that are similarly relaxing and fun, is essential to make sense of life when working in a high-pressure environment. This chapter presents some examples of how individuals might react under stress and then discusses how these individuals might react in a more self-affirming way. The chapter also presents coping strategies from the literature that are generally helpful in dealing with stress.

## SARAH'S STORY

Sarah graduated 3 months previously from her nursing degree. The motto for the Short-Stay Unit where Sarah works is "fast paced and patient turnover." The patient population usually consists of patients who have surgical procedures performed and need to be monitored for 24 to 48 hours postoperatively. This story tells what happened to her on her first day after orientation, when she was given her own patient assignment. The assignment included two thyroidectomy patients, two laparoscopic cholecystectomy patients, and a young man who had had an appendectomy. The night nurse reported that all her patients had an uneventful night. As Sarah was getting started on her rounds, the call light went off in one of the thyroidectomy patients' rooms. The patient was complaining of difficulty breathing. He was extremely restless and said that he could not get enough air. There was a strange sound as he breathed in. Sarah guessed that he was having inspiratory stridor, but Sarah had never heard this sound before in a real patient. She examined his thyroidectomy dressing site and noted a hematoma the size of a golf ball. Her heart was pounding in her chest, and she thought, what should she do? She knew she needed to get help *straight away*. Her hands were shaking so much that she could barely hold the phone to activate the rapid response team. She raised the head of the bed and put on the oxygen cannula. Almost immediately, help from the unit arrived, as well as the rapid response team. Sarah telephoned the surgeon and gave him the assessment information. The patient's respiratory status continued to deteriorate. The rapid response team leader called a code. The code response physician intubated the patient's airway with considerable difficulty. The surgeon arrived and the patient was whisked off to the operating room for emergency exploratory surgery and decompression of the hematoma. Sarah then made a call to the patient's wife and told her of the incident and that her husband was now in the operating room having emergency surgery. The wife was hysterical on the phone and Sarah was unsure of what to tell her and how to comfort her.

By this time, Sarah's knees were shaking so badly that she could barely stand and she felt like she was going to faint.

This experience made Sarah question whether she was cut out to work on this type of unit. This patient could have died and Sarah was not sure if she wanted that responsibility on her hands. This was her first emergency situation and she was aware that she was not sure what to do. She was worried about having the responsibility for people and making incorrect decisions that might affect their lives. After this experience, she dreaded going to work. She tried not to overthink about the experience and the situation, but she could not seem to stop. Sarah just could not relax. She was even dreaming about caring for patients and agonizing over what decisions she should make.

## COPING WITH STRESS IN NURSING

Sarah is anxious and fearful. Like other new nurses, her confidence in her knowledge and skills was waning. Confidence typically wanes during the first 6 months after graduation (Chernomas, Care, McKenzie, Guse, & Currie, 2010), so finding ways to feel supported, comforted, and buoyant are essential when beginning nursing practice. Stressors are a reality of demanding careers and thus it is important to be aware of coping strategies that are useful in the long term, and healthy for mind and body.

A previous chapter (Chapter 6, Appraising and Moderating Stressful Situations) explored the notion that the way individuals react to stress may depend on how they appraise the stressor. It also considered the tendency to use habits of coping that have been acquired serendipitously through life and which may not be used with intention or mindfulness. Folkman (2013) also explains that there are different types of coping behaviors and each of them can be useful or helpful in their own way at different times. What matters, however, is that they are used judiciously and with conscious intent. Therefore, it is useful to summarize them briefly (Table 11.1). Problem-focused coping is when the stressor is faced, and there are attempts to resolve it. Emotion-focused coping is when there are attempts to minimize or moderate the emotional reaction to the stressor. Maladaptive coping is when unconscious habits of mind are resorted to in an effort to make the stressor go away without ever having to directly face it. Sometimes these maladaptive styles

Table 11.1 Types of Coping

| Problem-Focused Coping | Emotion-Focused Coping | Maladaptive Coping |
|---|---|---|
| The stressor is faced with an aim of resolving it, through:<br>• Information seeking<br>• Assistance to manage<br>• Removing oneself | Rather than manage the situation, the aim is to moderate the emotional reaction by:<br>• Meditation<br>• Talking to a confidante<br>• Journaling<br>• Positive self-talk<br>• Reframing<br>• Recognizing cognitive distortions | Rather than manage the situation or the emotion, the aim is to avoid the stressor, and acts may be unconscious such as:<br>• Rumination, reliving<br>• Numbness and dissociation<br>• Displacement<br>• Avoidance and disengagement |

are triggered in times of extreme crisis and designed to protect the mind from overwhelming distress, but when they are used to deal with everyday stressors they can interfere with work and social functioning. For example, if a nurse coped with the stress of dealing with anxious patients by displacing her own anxiety onto those very patients, the nurse would not be a safe practitioner. Nor would the nurse be suited to the profession. Becoming conscious of the kinds of coping strategies used in a stressful situation is important. So, too, is widening one's repertoire of coping choices.

This chapter concentrates on the emotion-focused realm, offering strategies to building supportive relationships, meditation, embracing your spiritual life, pet therapy, volunteering, and using music, humor, and exercise.

*Responding effectively to stress is one of the most challenging experiences for nurses. Learning how to consciously apply coping mechanisms is the key. Otherwise, you may find yourself simply reacting to, and thus vulnerable to, the pressures of nursing work.*

## Building Supportive Relationships

Building professional and nonprofessional relationships is vital in establishing a support system. Support systems provide different options for guidance and emotional support.

### Colleagues

Building positive, nurturing relationships with colleagues provide a safe haven for letting off emotional steam. Connecting with colleagues provides opportunities to relate, vent about stressful situations, and reaffirm that a nurse is not alone in dealing with the trials and tribulations of the work environment. Just being able to talk to someone who "walks in your shoes" and who can relate to the situation helps to work through stress and frustrations. Colleagues with more experience can provide guidance and insights into challenging situations and can explore positive solutions. Finding a trusted professional colleague with whom to share experiences also provides a nurturing relationship for that person as well.

### Pam's Story

Pam knows having a support person is very important. She works in a pediatric cancer unit. Just dealing with the emotional aspects of this type of work is very stressful. Pam feels lucky because she found a friend on the unit that she can confide in. At the end of the day, she can call her friend and talk about how the day went. Pam feels that her friend understands what she is going through since she works on the same unit and experiences the same situations that Pam does. As a result, they have developed a bond. Pam does not know what she would have done as a new graduate nurse if she did not find a friend like Susan to lean on.

Nurses can build their professional support system by connecting with social networks such as professional nursing organizations and nursing listservs. The bottom line in this is finding a support system that works for the individual concerns and provides the right outlet that allows for refilling what could be called the "emotional bucket." A list of nursing community websites that may be useful:

- AllNurses: allnurses.com
- American Nurses Association: www.nursingworld.org/ana
- Australian College of Nursing: www.acn.edu.au

- Canadian Nurses Association: www.cna-aiic.ca
- International Council of Nurses: www.icn.ch
- National Student Nurses Association: www.nsna.org
- Royal College of Nursing: www.rcn.org.uk

### Family and Friends

Nurses also need to develop support systems outside of the work environment. Being able to vent to a neutral person who does not have an investment in the work under consideration provides a "sounding board" for bouncing off ideas in a nonthreatening manner. Support from family and friends helps validate an individual and grounds that person back into his or her personal values and beliefs. Connecting with family and friends provides a sense of belonging and reaffirms the nurse's sense of self-worth. Just sitting with a friend, enjoying a cup of tea, coffee, or hot chocolate or a cool drink, visiting with a family member, or attending a social event, helps rejuvenate emotional health. Just knowing that family and friends can be leaned on in times of stressful situations provides a solid foundation for coping with life's challenges.

*"I came from a big family who lived together on a farm in rural Virginia. As farmers, we relied on each other for everything—food, clothing, and shelter. I always felt crowded in the farmhouse having to share a room with my three brothers and I couldn't wait to move up to the city for nursing school. Then I took a job in the ICU and it wasn't very long before I realized just how important they were to me and how much I missed just being with them. I was really glad when texting was invented. Now, we email and text all the time." (Brad)*

## Meditation

Meditation can be used as a way to increase calmness and physical relaxation, improve psychological balance, or enhance overall wellness. Meditation focuses an individual's attention so that the person is mindful of his or her thoughts, feelings, and sensations and is able to observe them in a nonjudgmental way. Using meditation allows for the flow of emotions and thoughts to be controlled and helps concentrate on day-to-day activities. Meditation has several health benefits, such as reducing blood pressure, relaxing muscles, reducing anxiety, and eliminating stressful thoughts. Meditation also helps meditators to learn to "stay in the moment" and connect with themselves, known as *centering*. Centering allows meditators to focus on the "here and now" and provides them with time to calmly rejuvenate their mind (Gutierrez, Fox, & Wood, 2015).

Meditation does not have to be a religious activity. There are many styles of meditation, but all have four common elements.

- Select a quiet location. Many meditators prefer a quiet place with as few distractions as possible, which can be particularly helpful for beginners. People who have been practicing meditation for a longer period sometimes develop the ability to meditate in public places, like waiting rooms or buses.
- Choose a specific and comfortable posture. Depending on the type being practiced, meditation can be done while sitting, lying down, standing, walking, or in other specific positions.
- Focus your attention. Focusing one's attention is usually a part of meditation. For example, the meditator may focus on a mantra (a specially chosen word or set of words), an object, or simply the rise and fall of the breath.
- Have an open attitude. An open attitude during meditation means letting distractions come and go naturally without stopping to think about them. When distracting or wandering thoughts occur, they are not suppressed; instead, the meditator gently brings attention back to the focus. In some types of meditation, the meditator learns to observe the rising and falling of thoughts and emotions as they spontaneously occur.

## Spirituality

### Nancy's Story

Nancy found working in a hospice facility very difficult. She dealt with terminally ill patients on a daily basis. Nancy feels that if she did not have her faith and spirituality to fall back on, she would not be able to renew herself each day in order to return to work. Nancy confided in her friend, "I know there is a higher power that is looking over my shoulder and guiding me in caring for my patients. I pray each night to give me strength to care for my patients and help them deal with their end-of-life issues."

Like Nancy, some nurses find considerable support in their faith and spirituality. Spirituality is defined as a "basic or inherent quality in all humans that involves a belief in something greater than the self and a faith that positively affirms life" (Miller, 1995, p. 257). Spirituality provides a way to explore finding meaning and purpose in life and how that meaning relates to oneself, as well as family and community. Finding purpose and meaning in life leads to a sense of fulfillment. Nurses find that when they are more aware of their own spirituality, they are able to help and care for their patients and families in a more holistic way. Through spirituality, nurses are able to retain some balance in their life and put stressful situations into a perspective that allows them to move on (Ablett & Jones, 2007; Tugade & Fredrickson, 2004; Tusaie & Dyer, 2004).

## Pets as Healers

Building support systems such as making friends at work and using meditation to reduce job stress has been discussed. Now this chapter shifts to other sources of comfort. A large body of literature supports the role of pets in promoting health and well-being (Garrity, Stallones, Marx, & Johnson, 1989; Kidd & Kidd, 1985; McNicholas & Collis, 2006; Wells, 2007). Although causal associations between companion animal ownership and the alleviation of symptoms of specific diseases have not been definitively shown (Wells, 2009), it is a widely held belief in Western culture that pets are a good source of social support and may, in fact, be healers in their own right. Ask any pet owner and they will affirm this.

### Mary's Story

When Mary was a new graduate, she had a Maltese cross dog, Pete, who used to go everywhere with her that she was allowed to take him. She would have taken him to work if she could have because he really earned the title of "best friend." Mary used to come home exhausted from the emergency department but, no matter how tired she was, she knew she needed to take Pete for a walk and then feed him. And no matter how cranky she was, Pete always greeted her so enthusiastically, that she felt as though she was the most wonderful person in the world. They would walk and then go home and sit by the fire and Mary would tell her dog about her day. Pete would listen attentively for about 10 minutes and then he would yawn and that was Mary's signal to put it behind her and do the other things she needed, or wanted, to do.

But what can a nurse do if they do not have a pet, or cannot have one because of housing restrictions or allergies? Although companion dogs and cats are the most common pets, many people enjoy the calming effect of watching fish in an aquarium or having a small caged pet such as a guinea pig. Simply interacting with friends' pets can also be restful. Someone without pets can also offer to pet-sit when they are away, or want a day out, or can simply make a point of holding and petting animals when visiting with friends.

## Volunteering

### Kate's Story

Kate works in a high-pressure intensive care unit and when she comes home from work, she is usually too tired to think of anything but sleep. But every Sunday morning, Kate has trained herself to go to church and teach a Sunday school class. She finds that working with small children who are excited to hear the Bible stories she tells them is so energizing that she remembers that there is more to life than people dying.

Volunteer activities can reduce stress by helping to refocus one's attention from the problems and concerns at work to making a contribution to a worthy organization. Many organizations like local animal shelters, shelters for sufferers of domestic violence, or churches or other local groups that feed older adults or the homeless are rarely sufficiently staffed or funded. They will usually be grateful of an offer to help for a day, a week, or a weekend, or one day a week. Some groups such as domestic violence shelters have training requirements, while others will take any help they can get. Most prefer to have someone commit to a specific schedule.

An exciting opportunity for nursing students in many programs is to volunteer their services to poor and other needy communities, both in their own countries and abroad. The staff members who accompany them speak of the richness of the experience for volunteer nurses in the communities in which their students work (de Chesnay, 2005). Welch (2009) wrote about her extensive volunteer activities on medical missions to Central America in terms of how rewarding it was to spend time in a community and get to know the people. Even the smallest intervention can make a huge difference in people's lives.

## Music

Music has been a basic part of human life in every culture throughout history. Oliver Wendell Holmes (1809–1894), the American author and physician, advised of the health value of immersion in music: "Take a music bath once or twice a week for a few seasons. You will find it is to the soul what a water bath is to the body" (Dholakia, n.d). During the Crimean War, Florence Nightingale was a proponent of careful consideration of all environmental needs of patients, including music to aid in healing. Music therapy has been provided for patients for many years and has been found to provide physical as well as emotional benefits. In a study of university students, it has been found that simply listening to music reduced subjective levels of stress, and when the students were told that relaxation was the reason for the music listening, both subjective and objective evidence (lower cortisol and alpha-amylase levels) of stress reduction were noted (Linnemann, Ditzen, Strahler, Doerr, & Nater, 2015). Studies exploring the effect of music on well-being is a growing field and has numerous applications, particularly if personal music preferences and the context of care are taken into account (Terry, Curran, & Karageorghis, 2014).

Music is a mode of self-care that is very individual in terms of preference but is a universal soother. After the busy work shift is over, music can be a safe haven of self-care. As Maya Angelou (1974) describes, taking refuge in music can be a way of relieving stress and playing or listening to music, or singing, can provide respite from the stresses of the day. Some have described the feeling of playing music as a physical sensation and the creative feeling of making an art piece. The detachment from other thoughts provides a mental resting time. Whether playing, singing, or listening, the use of music for relaxation and unwinding is an excellent option to cope with stress.

## Humor and Laughter

### Robert's Story

Robert knew that working in the busiest emergency department (ED) in the city has its stresses. It is never known who or what is coming in the door. One minute the ED is quiet and the next minute chaos has erupted. Patients with gunshot wounds, traumatic injuries from car accidents, heart attacks, and strokes are just a few types of cases he sees every day. Some days, he does not even get to take a break or eat his lunch. Working in this type of environment, Robert has learned to add humor and laughter into his life. It helps him relieve his stress and keeps him grounded in the simple things in life. He really likes going to the comedy club after work on weekends. A group of colleagues from the ED go together and they just have a great time laughing and cutting up. Robert can tell that this stress outlet helps him to cope with the demands of working in the ED.

There is an old saying, "laughter is the best medicine," but this is an idea that is actually borne out in clinical research. Studies have shown that humor and laughter has many benefits, including strengthening the immune system (Savage, Lujan, Thipparthi, & DiCarlo, 2017), relieving stress, and anxiety (Abel & Maxwell, 2002; Iwasaki, MacKay, & Mactavish, 2005) and reducing postoperative pain (Elmali & Akpinar, 2017). Studies have also shown that introducing humor and a playful culture into the work environment increases workers' focus on tasks and achievements (Cheng & Wang, 2015).

The movie, *Patch Adams* (Shadyac, 1989), portrayed the life of Hunter "Patch" Adams, MD. Adams was one of the first medical practitioners to discuss the value of incorporating therapeutic humor and laughter into his bedside routine in caring for his patients. Thanks to his innovative actions, clowning has become a common complementary therapy used in many medical contexts, from very young children to the older age groups, all over the world, and studies have shown that it reduces anxiety and increases treatment compliance (Meiri, Ankri, Hamad-Saied, Konopnicki, & Pillar, 2016), reduces pain perception (Kocherov et al., 2016), and improves quality of life in gerontology settings (Lelièvre et al., 2018).

There is now strong evidence suggesting that laughter and humor can be effective in promoting well-being in a whole range of populations and contexts, including nursing, however, it is vital to remember that what an individual finds funny is a personal taste and response, and it requires judicious use (Tremayne, 2014). Nurses and student nurses often experience or participate in black humor, sometimes referred to as aberrant or gallows humor, during stressful or difficult situations in the workplace. This as an emotion-focused coping technique. The term "gallows humor" was first coined by Sigmund Freud in his theory of humor (1905/1960). Freud believed that individuals use joking as a method to relieve anxiety and stress when dealing with feelings of pain, fear, and horror; however, the use of gallows humor may seem inappropriate to others. What is funny to one group of healthcare providers may not be amusing to another group (Bennett, 2003).

Despite this word of caution, humor and laughter are a joyous coping strategy and there are many sources of it. It is important to begin to look for opportunities that can bring humor and laughter into life—watching comedies on television or at the movies, drawing pictures with young children, reading comics or humorous novels, or going to a comedy club.

### Exercise to Energize

"Those who think they have not time for bodily exercise will sooner or later have to find time for illness" (Edward Stanley, Earl of Derby, 1978). Frequently, new graduates find stress relief by blogging their thoughts. The following is an online blog from a new graduate:

OK...think!...get the blood cultures from the central line and log them in to the computer. Whose IV pump is beeping? Uh oh ... That lady doesn't look like she did early this morning ... maybe she needs some oxygen. Oh no! Her O2 sats are 88%. Do something! Now the sweet elderly man in 816 wants some tea for his wife. Just a minute, I'll be right there. There goes that IV alarm again! It's 10:30 already and I haven't even given meds. Think! What's next? It goes on and on ... I'm just feeling so stupid today ... like I don't know how to do anything ... 1 pm and I am stressed. I swallow my sandwich in 10 minutes still wondering if I'll ever get finished today ... and I glance outside at the sunshine. A quick walk in the sun, deep breathing, and stretching. It just took 20 minutes and it is amazing how much clearer my head is. What is it about just walking that does that to a person? Endorphins? Fresh air? The hospital has an inside walking track too – convenient. It's been the only a few weeks but I'm finding that a 20- or 30-minute walk right after work is what I crave to clear my head and ready myself for going home at the end of the day. And I feel so much better – like things aren't as bad as they were when I started walking. (Barbara Jean, new graduate, RN)

It is difficult to imagine that anyone would suggest that more exercise after an exhausting day of caring for patients would be helpful. Wasn't that *enough* exercise already? Not really. During each day, nurses go through enough activation of their stress responses to completely deplete their bodies; physical resources via increased muscle tension, increased heart and respiratory rates and blood pressure, and the chemical reactions brought on by the stresses of the job each day. With the competing demands for attention and the associated emotions on the job, a nurse's reservoir of coping strategies will probably run dry after a busy shift. Physical exercise is a key factor in managing your stress and building personal resilience.

The physical and emotional benefits of exercise have been well documented over many years (Centers for Disease Control and Prevention, 2009). The biochemicals (serotonin, dopamine, and endorphins) that produce a feeling of well-being, the tension reducing and cathartic effects of aerobic exercise, and the overall improvements in energy and cognitive functioning are but a few examples of the benefits. Exercise is the most efficient and effective method of burning up the tensions of the day. Many publications since the 1960s have also noted improved health and well-being for individuals who exercise regularly. In more recent years, cost-reduction benefits related to decreased employee sick time, injuries, and absenteeism have been demonstrated, and many healthcare organizations have begun offering onsite exercise and wellness facilities (Powers & Howley, 2014). But exercise does not have to be in an expensive facility. If a healthcare institution does not have an onsite gym or pool, there are other opportunities. Exploring the type of exercise that best suits as a coping strategy is a first move. A 20-minute walk or jog after work is an excellent time to decelerate thoughts while gaining physical benefits. Some prefer dancing or gym classes for the added companionship and motivation. Whether taken alone or in a group, moderate or vigorous, regular activity and exercise is also essential for caretakers to take care of themselves (Table 11.2).

One sport that is becoming popular in the nursing world (particularly in the United States, Canada, Australia, and New Zealand) for recreation and exercise is called *geocaching* (pronounced *geo-cashing*). Played with global positioning system (GPS) devices, this treasure hunting game covers 192 countries throughout the world. The point is to locate hidden treasure containers outdoors and then share the

Table 11.2 Exercises for Sustained Performance Benefits

| Moderate Intensity Exercises | Vigorous Intensity Exercises |
| --- | --- |
| Water aerobics | Swimming laps |
| Walking briskly | Tai chi |
| Bicycling | Aerobic dancing |
| Tennis (doubles) | Jogging/running |
| Ballroom dancing | Walking briskly |
| General gardening | Heavy gardening |
| | Jumping rope |
| | Hiking uphill or with a heavy backpack |

Source: Adapted from the U.S. Department of Health and Human Services (2008).

experiences online. The treasure is usually something inexpensive and fun. From coins to stories, finding such treasures becomes a delight for those who participate in the hunt, while hiding the treasures offers additional entertainment. The activity gets participants outdoors and walking, the treasure hunt is fun and participants worldwide can join.

Beginning exercise soon after the shift ends is important. Frequently after a busy shift, getting caught up in the multiple things that have to be done is easy (cooking, shopping, washing, and the like) and it is tempting to skip exercise, and this omission can become habitual. It is important to think of exercise time as "me time" that provides respite from the work life and is a healthy transition into your personal life.

## Other Relaxing Activities

There is really no end to the kind of activities that can be used to de-stress. It is a matter of each person finding what works and then that person making a commitment to engage in the activity on a regular basis. It is essential to develop a routine—both at work and for fun after work. A few more ideas are: gardening or sewing; making jewelry; collecting shells, books, antiques, or anything else; reading; attending art and museum exhibitions, plays, concerts, and movies;

as well as blogging and using Facebook, MySpace, and Twitter. Joining a club or a class that is not related to work is also very relaxing. This could be a cooking class, book club, sports group, or language or writing class.

## SARAH'S STORY REVISITED

To revisit Sarah's story from the beginning of the chapter, as time went on, Sarah developed a support system by building a relationship with her preceptor. This gave Sarah an outlet to vent her frustrations and stresses with her job at work, and she finds she is able to cope more effectively with the day-to-day pressures as a new graduate nurse. The preceptor is a seasoned nurse with a decade of experience who encourages Sarah to look at the positive impact she has on her patients' lives as well as assists her with what she still needs to learn.

Sarah engages in other strategies to relieve the pressures from work. She has found she enjoys taking walks in the park in her neighborhood after work. Walking gives her time to reflect on the positive aspects of her life and to walk off the tension that sometimes occurs from her work situation. Another strategy that Sarah uses to reconnect to life and regain a work–life balance is to invite friends over on weekends to play cards. Connecting with other individuals outside of work provides her time to focus on these relationships and allows her to reconnect with the world around her.

## CONCLUSION

Nurses will likely experience a myriad of emotions and feelings in addition to fatigue while working. Many new graduates express feelings of being overloaded, without enough time to complete the things that they need to accomplish. They can feel distress about patients, their conditions, and life situations; and then compare themselves to coworkers who appear to be so much more competent and in control. This may lead to feelings of frustration and self-doubt and this combination can be a perfect recipe for burnout. To best help patients, nurses must practice self-care and find an appropriate balance between their work lives and their personal lives. Nurses did not join the profession to be martyrs, yet it is difficult to flip the switch to turn off the nurse mode and begin focusing on oneself.

There are, however, various methods of re-entering the personal world after leaving the work world. Finding an activity or means of leaving work behind and managing life outside of work is a task for everyone who practices nursing. Finding a combination that fits personal preferences and personality and offers the needed refreshment is important. Intentional and regular separation from the work world keeps nurses healthier and more satisfied with nursing practice.

## LEARNING ACTIVITIES

Select one of the activities from the following list to experience meditation or a form of spirituality. Try the activity for a week or two and note the effect that this activity has on your stress levels. If you wish, share your experiences via a blog, email, or tweet, or just discuss them with your fellow students.

1. Attend a local yoga class.
2. Sign up for a local meditation class.
3. Attend a religious service or a Bible study class at your church.
4. Find a quiet place, play some soft music, dim the lights, and relax for 30 minutes.
5. Organize a small group of friends or fellow students to try these activities for humor and laughter:
   - Watch the movie *Patch Adams*.
   - Go to a comedy club with a group of friends.
   - Go to the store or library and buy or borrow a book from the humor section.
   - Take a child to an amusement park.

## REFERENCES

Abel, M. H., & Maxwell, D. (2002). Humor and affective consequences of a stressful task. *Journal of Social and Clinical Psychology, 21*(2), 165–191. doi:10.1521/jscp.21.2.165.22516

Ablett, J. R., & Jones, R. S. P. (2007). Resilience and well-being in palliative care staff: A qualitative study of hospice nurses' experience of work. *Psycho-Oncology, 16*(8), 733–740. doi:10.1002/pon.1130

Angelou, M. (1974). *Gather together in my name*. New York, NY: Random House.

Bennett, H. J. (2003). Humor in medicine: Humor and health. *Southern Medical Journal, 96*(12), 1257–1261. doi:10.1097/01.SMJ.0000066657.70073.14

Centers for Disease Control and Prevention. (2009). *Physical activity.* Retrieved from https://www.cdc.gov/healthyweight/physical_activity/

Cheng, D., & Wang, L. (2015). Examining the energizing effects of humor: The influence of humor on persistence behavior. *Journal of Business and Psychology, 30*(4), 759–772. doi:10.1007/s10869-014-9396-z

Chernomas, W. M., Care, W. D., McKenzie, J. A., Guse, L., & Currie, J. (2010). "Hit the ground running": Perspectives of new nurses and nurse managers on role transition and integration of new graduates. *Nursing Leadership, 22*(4), 70–86. doi:10.12927/cjnl.2010.21598

de Chesnay, M. (2005). Teaching nurses about vulnerable populations. In M. de Chesnay (Ed.), *Caring for the vulnerable: Perspectives in nursing theory, practice and research* (pp. 349–356). Sudbury, MA: Jones & Bartlett.

Dholakia, C. (n.d). *Inspiration: An EBook featuring 1001 inspiring quotes.* Retrieved from http://www.icosvietnam.com/wp-content/uploads/2018/11/inspiration.pdf

Elmali, H., & Akpinar, R. B. (2017). The effect of watching funny and unfunny videos on postsurgical pain levels. *Complementary Therapies in Clinical Practice, 26*, 36–41. doi:10.1016/j.ctcp.2016.11.003

Folkman, S. (2013). Stress: Appraisal and coping. In M. Gellman & J. Turner (Eds.), *Encyclopedia of behavioral medicine* (pp. 1913–1915). New York, NY: Springer.

Garrity, T., Stallones, L., Marx, M. B., & Johnson, T. (1989). Pet ownership and attachment as supportive factors in the health of the elderly. *Anthrozoos, 3*(1), 35–44. doi:10.2752/089279390787057829

Gutierrez, D., Fox, J., & Wood, A. W. (2015). Center, light, and sound: The psychological benefits of three distinct meditative practices. *Counseling and Values, 60*(2), 234–247. doi:10.1002/cvj.12016

Iwasaki, Y., MacKay, K., & Mactavish, J. (2005). Gender-based analyses of coping with stress among professional managers: Leisure coping and non-leisure coping. *Journal of Leisure Research, 37*(1), 1–28. doi:10.1080/00222216.2005.11950038

Kidd, A. H., & Kidd, R. M. (1985). Children's attitudes toward their pets. *Psychology Reports, 57*(11), 15–31. doi:10.2466/pr0.1985.57.1.15

Kocherov, S., Hen, Y., Jaworowski, S., Ostrovsky, I., Eidelman, A. I., Gozal, Y., & Chertin, B. (2016). Medical clowns reduce pre-operative anxiety, post-operative pain and medical costs in children undergoing outpatient penile surgery: A randomised controlled trial. *Journal of Paediatrics and Child Health, 52*(9), 877–881. doi:10.1111/jpc.13242

Lelièvre, A., Gérard, S., Hermabessière, S., Martinez, M., Péran, B., & Rolland, Y. (2018). Humour therapy, laughter and the intervention of clowns in gerontology. *Soins Gerontologie, 23*(130), 37–43. doi:10.1016/j.sger.2018.01.008

Linnemann, A., Ditzen, B., Strahler, J., Doerr, J. M., & Nater, U. M. (2015). Music listening as a means of stress reduction in daily life. *Psychoneuroendocrinology, 60*, 82–90. doi:10.1016/j.psyneuen.2015.06.008

McNicholas, J., & Collis, G. M. (2006). Animals as social supports: Insights for understanding animal assisted therapy. In A. Fine (Ed.), *Handbook on animal-assisted therapy: Theoretical foundations and guidelines for practice* (pp. 49–71). Amsterdam, The Netherlands: Elsevier.

Meiri, N., Ankri, A., Hamad-Saied, M., Konopnicki, M., & Pillar, G. (2016). The effect of medical clowning on reducing pain, crying, and anxiety in children aged 2–10 years old undergoing venous blood drawing—A randomized controlled study. *European Journal of Pediatrics, 175*(3), 373–379. doi:10.1007/s00431-015-2652-z

Miller, M. A. (1995). Culture, spirituality, and women's health. *Journal of Obstetric, Gynecologic, and Neonatal Nursing, 24*(3), 257–263. doi:10.1111/j.1552-6909.1995.tb02471.x

Powers, S. K., & Howley, E. T. (2014). *Exercise physiology: Theory and application to fitness and performance.* New York, NY: McGraw-Hill Humanities/Social Sciences/Languages.

Savage, B. M., Lujan, H. L., Thipparthi, R. R., & DiCarlo, S. E. (2017). Humor, laughter, learning, and health! A brief review. *Advances in Physiology Education, 41*(3), 341–347. doi:10.1152/advan.00030.2017

Shadyac, T. (1989). *Patch Adams* [motion picture]. Hollywood: Universal Pictures.

Stanley, E. (1978). *Disraeli, Derby, and the Conservative Party: Journals and memoirs of Edward Henry, Lord Stanley, 1849-1869.* Madison, WI: Harvester Press.

Terry, P. C., Curran, M., & Karageorghis, C. I. (2014). *Does music really make a difference? Meta-analytic review of a century of research.* Proceedings of the 28th International Congress of Applied Psychology (ICAP 2014). International Association of Applied Psychology (IAAP).

Tremayne, P. (2014). Using humour to enhance the nurse-patient relationship. *Nursing Standard, 28*(30), 37–40. doi:10.7748/ns2014.03.28.30.37.e8412

Tugade, M., & Fredrickson, B. (2004). Resilient individuals use emotions to bounce back from negative emotional experiences. *Journal of Personality and Social Psychology, 86*(2), 320–333. doi:10.1037/0022-3514.86.2.320

Tusaie, K., & Dyer, J. (2004). Resilience: A historical review of the construct. *Holistic Nursing Practice, 18*(1), 3–10. doi:10.1097/00004650-200401000-00002

Welch, V. (2009). Investing in the future: The value of volunteerism. *Urologic Nursing, 29*(4), 212–213.

Wells, D. L. (2007). Domestic dogs and human health: An overview. *British Journal of Health Psychology, 12*(1), 145–156. doi:10.1348/135910706X103284

Wells, D. L. (2009). Associations between pet ownership and self-reported health status in people suffering from chronic fatigue syndrome. *The Journal of Alternative and Complementary Medicine, 15*(4), 407–413. doi:10.1089/acm.2008.0496

# 12

# Leading a Resilient Nursing Workforce

## Linda Shields

### INTRODUCTION

Much has been written on theories of leadership and what makes a good leader. Recently, short courses and even entire postgraduate degrees that promise to train students to be leaders have proliferated. Lord Byron is well known for saying "when we think we lead we most are led" (Byron, 1821). While Byron was never known for his humility, such sentiments do indicate one essence of a good leader. Leadership theories have been around forever. The Bible is full of them, and quotes about leadership by ancient writers such as Lao-Tzu (Shun, 1995) and Homer (Taplin, 1986) are still commonly used. If one cannot name a dozen well-known leaders, then surely one needs to read more, and when curiosity can be almost immediately gratified through an Internet search, there is no excuse for not being able to name at least a few. This chapter is going to tell the stories of some people who have been (and still are) great leaders in nursing, as well as related various aspects of leadership theory.

Have I become a leader? I hope so, although others will be better able to judge that. In the following, I discuss some of the characteristics of a good leader as I understand them, and tell the stories of some wonderful leaders I have known, and what—in particular—makes them leaders. Most of these people will not make those the "most famous people" list, but they are leaders nonetheless. They are my nursing heroes.

## PROFESSOR ROGER WATSON

The International Council of Nurses (ICN) is the leading international body for nursing. For many years, it was led by Dr. Margretta Styles (Basu, 2005) who, as president, stated that, "Nursing will know it has succeeded when a nurse is awarded a Nobel Prize." As the Nobel Prize is the ultimate accolade for intellectual and cultural achievement, it is a laudable goal for nurses to strive toward. Roger Watson (Figure 12.1) is a modern leader who, as editor-in-chief of the *Journal of Advanced Nursing,* has seen the journal rise to its status as one of the top international journals in nursing. In response to the question of nurses winning the Nobel Prize, he has stated that this may prove difficult as nursing is such a hybrid of philosophies; there is no one agreed definition of nursing, and it is neither a uniquely scientific nor artistic endeavor (Watson, 2008). Nursing is made up of such a range of activities, theories, and constructs that it is hard to combine into a single entity. Hence, the Nobel Prize, which is awarded in specific disciplines such as medicine, science, or literature, may not be a good

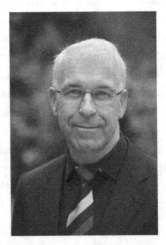

**Figure 12.1** Professor Roger Watson.

fit with nursing. Watson does, however, conclude that this should never preclude nurses from striving to win such accolades, and that personal enterprise and striving for the highest standards and goals should be an integral part of nurses' ethics and motivation.

*An important leadership strategy is to assert your own beliefs even if others may criticize you.*

Despite how powerfully he argued this case, many disagreed with Watson's remarks, and he received correspondence from other nurses that was unconstructive. Nevertheless, he showed great leadership in saying what he did, as this made nurses sit up, take notice, and reflect on the nature of nursing—what nursing is all about and each individual nurse's part in it. A willingness to put oneself in line for criticism and, more negatively, personal attack is a characteristic of a leader that I personally applaud and try to emulate (see also the University of Hull, 2018).

In 1990, Paul Keating, who was later to be the prime minister of Australia, said "Leadership is not about being nice. It's about being right and being strong" (Keating & National Press Club, 1990). Some leaders are less public than such political figures, but display characteristics that can endear and infuriate at the same time. While many strive to be seen as "nice" people, occasionally, there are some who lead by bringing issues to attention that, while they need to be addressed, may cause intense irritation. Such a leader was Sister Mary Dorothea.

## SISTER MARY DOROTHEA, RSM

The first time I met Sister Mary Dorothea, I saw an energetic woman, aged in her early 60s, who spoke in a strong, determined voice about what she expected of me as a new employee of her hospital. As a Sister of Mercy (Institute of the Sisters of Mercy, Australia, 2007), Sister Mary Dorothea had devoted her life to the care of children at the Mater Hospital, a large Catholic hospital in Brisbane, Australia (Shields, 1999). When I went to work there, Dot, as she was affectionately known, had been director of nursing (under the position's several titles) for many years. She had begun life in a small country town, completed her nursing "training" (as it was called in those days) at the Mater Hospital, and then joined the convent in 1938. She ruled with a fist of iron in a velvet glove. Her determination to make her hospital a family-friendly place for her small patients was matched only by her commitment to making it a safe, secure, and good place to work for her nurses. Dot knew all our names (even those who, like me, worked permanent night duty). She may not have known our children's names, but there was nothing she liked better than to take us aside and find out how they were getting on at school and, most importantly, she listened and remembered what we told her. Then, at our next encounter, she would ask salient questions about our families.

Working in a children's hospital is very rewarding but it can have its downsides. The death of a child is always distressing and, when this occurred on night duty, seemed to be even more so. One of my fondest memories of Dot (and the other nuns who worked with her) is indicative of the care she gave to her nursing staff. When a child was dying on the ward, we would, of course, support the parents to the best of our abilities. Dot and the two Sisters of Mercy who were her nursing supervisors (the term then used), Sister Marie and Sister Collette, would leave their beds, come into the ward, and make cups of tea and coffee for the nursing staff.

> *Another leadership strategy is to demonstrate care through compassionate action.*

As well as having so much compassion for her charges, Dot was a fighter, but always in the nicest way possible, and this encompassed her advocacy for children and their families. She was notorious among the hospital board for bringing her advocacy to the fore at the end of a discussion in an executive meeting. After a long discussion of some point about running the hospital, just when everyone thought a decision had been made, Dot would say "Ah, yes, but children are different" and the discussion would have to begin all over again.

I learned many things from Dot. First, that good manners can be assertiveness in another guise. Next, that determination about something one thinks is right will help one be assertive, and that advocacy for others, as well as for oneself, is an important part of a nurse's role. However, the most important lesson I learned from Dot was the value of compassion, and how it is important not just for the children, families, and patients who come to nurses for care, but for those with whom one works. This lesson of compassion is especially important if one is in a leadership or management role.

While Dot was a fighter at a time when resources were (relatively) plentiful, my next hero is a leader in a time when all available resources were being used to fight a war.

## DAME MAUD McCARTHY

Emma Maud McCarthy (Figure 12.2) was born in Sydney, Australia, in 1859, the first child in the large family of a prominent solicitor, and her maternal uncle was the chief justice of Victoria, Sir William àBeckett (McCarthy, 1986). In 1891, giving her age as 28 (she was over 30), Maud, as she was known, began her training as a nurse at The London Hospital in Whitechapel. Her probationer report describes her as "a lady," "wanting courage," and "needing more force of character" (The London Hospital, 1894). However, by 1894, she had been made Sister and, along with six other Sisters from The London Hospital, was chosen to go to the war in South Africa as part of Princess Alexandra's Military Nursing Contingent. She served there from 1899 to 1902, and was awarded the Royal Red Cross, and the Queen's and the King's Medals.

In 1902, Queen Alexandra's Imperial Military Nursing Service (QAIMNS) was formed (Piggott, 1990). With high standards of

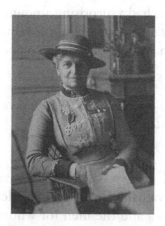

**Figure 12.2** Dame Maud McCarthy.

professional knowledge and experience required, these nurses were experts in modern nursing techniques. An inherent part of their work and training was to display a high level of compassion toward the servicemen whom they served. In 1903, Maud McCarthy joined QAIMNS as a matron, and served at the Royal Victoria Military Hospital Netley, then Millbank Military Hospital. In 1910, she was appointed a principal matron in the British War office.

When the First World War began in 1914, Maud McCarthy was promoted to matron-in-chief for France and Flanders. She left England on the first ship for the battlefields of the Western front, and was responsible for the administration of nursing facilities throughout the Somme campaign. Her authority covered nurses from Britain, Australia, Canada, New Zealand, South Africa, India, and the United States (Light, 2009). After the Armistice was signed on November 11, 1918, Maud McCarthy left France only after she had closed down her headquarters and ensured that all her nurses had arrived home safely. She remained matron-in-chief of QAIMNS and was decorated many times by the United Kingdom, France, Belgium, and the United States (McCarthy, 1986), including receiving the award of Dame Grand Cross.

After the war, Dame Maud McCarthy became matron-in-chief of the Territorial Army Nursing Service from 1920 to 1925. She was made a Lady of Grace of the Grand Priory of the Hospital of St. John of Jerusalem in England in 1919. Dame Maud died in 1949 in London. Sadly, now, in her own country, Australia, little is known about this great leader. She was much loved and respected by her nurses, by military confreres and commanders, and by her patients, with whom—given her lofty position—she had a surprising amount of interaction. Dame Maud McCarthy was a true leader, and it remains an indictment of Australian and British nursing that she is so poorly remembered.

*One key strategy you can take on is to promise to notice and validate nursing leaders you value.*

Dame Maud McCarthy was a great organizer and administrator, which, of course, are valuable qualities for leaders to possess. But her concern for her nurses and the men for whom they cared showed that under the tight military discipline, there lurked the same sort of compassion that Sister Mary Dorothea was able to demonstrate openly. My next hero had to hide all her compassion, ethics, and actions because her leadership put her life in danger on a daily basis.

## MARIA STROMBERGER

Maria Stromberger (Figure 12.3) was also active in wartime and, similarly to Dame Maud, she is not well remembered. Her leadership qualities had to be subtle and covert and draw no attention to her, and thus were very different from the other nurses described herein. Maria Stromberger was born in 1869 and, like Dame Maud, did not commence her nursing training until she was aged in her 30s (Benedict, 2006). While working in an infectious diseases hospital in Königshütte in Poland in 1942, she heard stories of terrible happenings at a Polish town called Auschwitz. Maria Stromberger, much to the disquiet of her sister, applied for, and got, the job as head nurse in the *Revier*, or camp hospital, for *Schutzstaffel* (SS) soldiers at Auschwitz. The *Revier* was in close proximity to the main crematorium and gas chambers, and so she saw and heard what was occurring there. She resolved that it was her humanitarian duty to try to help as many prisoners as she could. Until she herself became ill in 1944, Maria Stromberger smuggled in food, medicine, guns, and ammunition for the prisoners, and smuggled out letters, reports, and film of what was happening inside so that the world could be told of the horrors taking place there. Remarkably, she

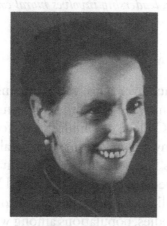

**Figure 12.3** Maria Stromberger.
*Source:* Published with permission of Archiv der Landeshauptstadt Bregenz.

was not caught—perhaps because she was highly intelligent as well as highly moral, as the consequences of being caught would have been not just death, but prolonged torture. Ironically, after the war she was imprisoned by the French who thought she was a Nazi, and it was not until Polish and Jewish prisoners and former members of the Polish Resistance presented testimony about her courageous work that she was freed (Benedict, 2006). Today, little is known about this woman who risked so much to help so many.

What life was like for Maria Stromberger is difficult to imagine, although after the war she never nursed again, choosing, instead, to work in a textile factory. The enormity of what she did deserves far more recognition than she has received, and her leadership qualities were of the highest order, particularly those surrounding moral choice, ethical actions, and being—and remaining—true to oneself and one's beliefs. Obviously, Maria Stromberger could receive no accolades for her work at the time in which she performed her momentous interventions, but that she is so little known now is sobering. Perhaps she personifies the humility characteristic of the greatest leaders.

While Maria Stromberger achieved much covertly, we now live in a world where many leadership achievements can be revealed openly. My next hero has been able to achieve much by leading people to work together, for the benefit of the nursing profession as a whole, and pediatric nursing in particular.

*Like ethical practice, leadership involves moral courage.*

## DR. JAN PRATT

Jan Pratt is a quiet achiever who, while nursing director of a large metropolitan community child health service, managed to bring into being the Australian College of Children and Young People's Nurses (2009a). As with many organizations in Australia, all the Australian states and territories had separate pediatric nursing organizations, some of which had been in place for decades. Historically, the separate states of Australia have been largely autonomous. They have distinct governing bodies, populations among whom rivalry has long existed (especially around that central Australian cultural entity, the sports team), and separate health systems. Pediatric nursing suffered from the state-related jingoism that was often a hamper to effective communication, with consequent negative effects on nursing as a profession and, ultimately, on patients and clients within the health services. Jan Pratt sought to change all that and, in the long term, improve care for children and families.

Such an endeavor was fraught with danger. Each Australian state thinks that its institutions do things better than the others, with traditions individual to each state, and the idea that each state is different. In 1979, Bob Hawke, who was prime minister from 1983 to 1991, said that Australia was the most over-governed country in the world, and this certainly was reflected in the number of pediatric nursing organizations. Jan was determined to join them together, to bring all pediatric (child health, adolescent, young people, neonatal, acute care, and so forth) nurses to a single table. Only by sundering the barriers between states, and by allowing a free exchange of ideas unhampered by artificial boundaries, would the health of children be best served, she believed.

In 2008, the Australian College of Children and Young People's Nurses was promulgated, with Dr. Jan Pratt as its first President (Australian College of Children and Young People's Nurses, 2009b). Not all the states have come on board, but Jan Pratt's quiet determination is continuing to influence the increasing professionalism of pediatric nursing in Australia. Jan Pratt's leadership attributes include a highly developed ability to break down communication barriers, to make people want to work with each other, to reflect on their own actions and abilities, and to question. One of her strongest leadership qualities is a quietly effective positive criticality, which she uses to promote people's awareness of their own actions and decisions.

*Some leaders are quiet achievers, enacting change by showing respect for others, self-belief, and never wavering from asking questions to produce reforms.*

## RESEARCH ON LEADERSHIP IN NURSING

The next part of this chapter focuses on how these individuals relate to the theories that have been developed around leadership. Leadership theories abound, with a recent Google search of "leadership characteristics" yielding over 65,000 hits. The International Council of Nurses has published a book on leadership for nurses, and they promote the following characteristics as necessary for what they term a "nurse leader: . . . vision and strategic thinking, external awareness, influence, motivation, confidence, trust, political skill, review, change and renewal of self and others, teamwork, partnerships and alliances" (Shaw, 2007, pp. 36–37), but there are variations on this.

A qualitative study of leadership in nurses in Sweden found several themes constituted good leadership: (a) to supply, meaning supply evidence, common space, and good structures for the work of nurses; (b) to support, that is to say, to be a role model, and to demonstrate appreciation and care of others; and (c) to shield, including being an advocate, to not tolerate unethical behavior, and to not be frightened of being critical (Gustafsson & Stenberg, 2017). A meta-ethnography of nursing leadership examined the question "What is caring in nursing leadership from the nurse leaders' perspective?" (Solbakken, Bergdahl, Rudolfsson, & Bondas, 2018, p. E3). They found six main themes: clinical presence that alleviates suffering; trust and respect; facilitated dialogue; confirmatory relations; strength and persistence; and being able to balance limited resources.

A relatively new concept of leadership is "clinical" leadership, and a plethora of definitions of this exist. Stanley and Stanley (2018) conducted a systematic literature review of clinical leadership, and found that while many definitions and concepts exist in the literature, in short, clinical leaders are those whose actions and interventions are in line with their values and beliefs. They are found at all levels in the nursing hierarchy, not just in management, executive levels, and so on, and in all clinical environments.

Certainly, my heroes have demonstrated the characteristics described in research, and I next explain what I personally see as the qualities and characteristics of a good leader and how these relate to my heroes.

## Courage

Some of the theorists and research in the preceding sections mention this quality. Maria Stromberger obviously had it very well developed. But how much courage did Roger Watson have to take the *Journal of Advanced Nursing* to the next level of development? Although no doubt exciting for him as a professional challenge, it also required considerable change. Additionally, competition from other highly regarded nursing journals that were much further developed than the *Journal of Advanced Nursing* was strong. Jan Pratt had to be very courageous when she challenged the traditionalists in the state-based pediatric nursing organizations and must have had many sleepless nights as a result. Although courage may not be something that can be learned, one can become *conditioned* to courage. Performing one brave act, sometimes (but not always) makes it easier to do another, and so on. However, many Victoria Cross winners, those whose bravery in battle has won them the highest of accolades, state that they do not regard themselves as particularly courageous. Rather, they attest that they acted on the spur of the moment when they saw others in trouble (Vasak, 2010).

## Willingness to Take Risks

This characteristic goes hand in hand with courage, and again, Maria Stromberger sits at the top of the list in clearly demonstrating this quality. She risked her life every day in Auschwitz. A good leader must be prepared to take a risk and celebrate—or suffer—the consequences. Not every risk will work out, and leaders must be able to pick themselves up, dust themselves off, and start all over again, as the song goes. Risks are, of course, not always of the magnitude that Maria Stromberger faced. For nurses today, risks are more often centered on the decisions made and the actions taken. But to never take a risk means nothing is ever tried, nothing is ever invented, nothing develops. Life would also be very boring without taking risks. Had Jan Pratt not taken a risk when she contacted pediatric nursing organizations in the other states, the Australian College of Children and Young People's Nurses would not have been created. A risk going wrong, or failing, can also provide the opportunity to learn from one's mistakes.

I once took a job in another country, and it turned out to be a really bad move for me personally. However, I learned a lot about that country and nursing in it. Most importantly, I learned about myself, as I found strengths I had not realized I possessed. While it was not very pleasant at the time, in retrospect, I would not have missed it for the world.

## Toughness

Some might refer to toughness as resilience, or determination, and perhaps it is a combination of those qualities. A leader of any kind has to be tough, but it is worth considering what that entails. Imagine the good feeling when you have persevered, know you are doing something right, and are determined that you are going to do the right thing. Dame Maud McCarthy had to be very tough to deal with the male officers of the time. The position of matron-in-chief had a significant amount of power and influence, but it is safe to assume that many men who, while they may never have come under her direct control, had to answer to her in other ways and were not always happy about doing so. One aspect of Dame Maud's command that is found repeatedly in reports and correspondence about her was her sustained advocacy for "her nurses." She felt a personal responsibility to ensure their safety and comfort while they were active frontline participants in the bloodiest conflict in history.

Determination is part of toughness, but it may not always be necessary to be tough when determination is called for. Perhaps being wily might be more appropriate: If a mountain cannot be climbed, then a way around it needs to be found.

## Making, and Learning From, Mistakes

In a radio broadcast I heard, a man who had been appointed director of a research facility funded by Bill Gates reported that Gates told him that if he was not making mistakes, then he wasn't doing his job. While I cannot locate this program to find this quotation, I have found one of Gates's other sayings: "Failure is a great teacher" (Gates, 2004). I am certain all of my heroes have made many mistakes, but their leadership is exemplified in the way that they persisted and succeeded, both despite these errors, and due to having learned from them.

## Tolerance and Celebration of Difference

The world is a much smaller place today than it was for Dame Maud or Maria Stromberger, or even for Sister Mary Dorothea. Today, travel to most other countries is relatively safe and simple.

Also, the mass media provides many opportunities to learn about other people and places from easily digestible forms of information. This should have led to more tolerance, and perhaps it has, and this is important as tolerance was sadly lacking in the world when Maria Stromberger was nursing. As leaders, nurses are well placed to celebrate difference because people of all races and creeds come to them for care; in fact, nurses are some of the most fortunate human beings because of our ability to help others. Tolerance and an awareness of the needs of others are surely characteristics of a good leader. Perhaps all nurses are leaders as these qualities are inherent in nursing.

### Compassion

A good leader who is aware of the needs of others must also be compassionate. Sister Mary Dorothea and her confreres in the Sisters of Mercy were, as the name of their order suggested, compassionate women. Dot had a highly developed ability to be touched by the children in her care, and never wavered in her dogged determination to ensure they received the very best care. Her compassion for both the children in her care and their families was the driving force in her life. Dot retired just at the time when HIV/AIDS was emerging and, driven by the compassion that was such a part of her calling, she left the children's hospital and set up a care home for young men with HIV/AIDS when others in the community were frightened by the disease and of those who suffered from it.

### Humility

To describe humility, I present the following pairs of leaders who were roughly contemporaries of each other: Jesus Christ and Tiberius Caesar; Thomas Jefferson and Napoleon Bonaparte; Mahatma Gandhi and Winston Churchill; Nelson Mandela and Margaret Thatcher. All have been great leaders, but those with humility—Christ, Jefferson, Gandhi, and Mandela—are, in my opinion, the greatest. All my nursing hero leaders have this defining quality, but Dot providing cups of tea for the nurses who were supporting the parents of a dying child perhaps best exemplifies humility in practice. Unless a leader has humility, he or she cannot lead effectively.

## CONCLUSION

*Courage, willingness to take risks, toughness, making and learning from mistakes, tolerance and celebration of difference, compassion and humility—these are qualities you can develop to empower your practice.*

Leadership is about, and focused on, others—after all, who does a leader lead if not other individuals? Nurses are in an ideal situation to lead others but nursing itself needs good leaders within the profession. To be a good leader, one needs vision, strategic thinking, motivation, confidence and determination, trust, political skill, courage and a willingness to take risks, strength, an ability to reflect on—and learn from—mistakes, compassion and, most important, humility. The examples presented here, those whose lives were spent as leaders in the service of others—Dame Maud McCarthy, Maria Stromberger, and Sister Mary Dorothea, RSM—and those who are nursing leaders today Roger Watson and Jan Pratt display special qualities that have enabled them to motivate, encourage, support, and, at times, succor, other nurses. This is important as, without leaders, nursing will not, as a profession or as a collection of human individuals, move forward. I believe that every reader of this book is either a potential or an existing leader.

### LEARNING ACTIVITIES

1. Interview someone you think is a very good leader in nursing. Record the interview and write it up as a paper for a nursing journal. Contextualize their work in terms of adding commentary on the leadership qualities you see in this person that you would wish to emulate.

2. Find classes on leadership at your local university, or online, in schools other than nursing (e.g., in a business school). Ask if you can attend on a casual basis to learn what other disciplines regard as leadership qualities.

3. Start a discussion group at your workplace. Seek permission if you need to, book a room, send out email messages with the topic (pick one in which you are really interested), and then guide the discussion around it.

# REFERENCES

Australian College of Children and Young People's Nurses. (2009a). Promoting excellence in health care for children and young people. Retrieved from http://www.accypn.org.au

Australian College of Children and Young People's Nurses. (2009b). Board members. Retrieved from http://www.accypn.org.au/members-area/governance-information/board

Basu, J. (2005). *Former UCSF Nursing Dean Margretta Styles dies at age 75*. UCSF News Office, San Francisco. Retrieved from http://news.ucsf.edu/releases/former-ucsf-nursing-dean-margretta-styles-dies-at-age-75

Benedict, S. (2006). Maria Stromberger: A nurse in the Resistance in Auschwitz. *Nursing History Review, 14*, 189–202. doi:10.1891/1062-8061.14.189

Byron, G. G. (Lord) (1821). *The Two Foscari*. Act II, Sc.1, p. 63. London: John Murray.

Gates, W. (2004). *Advancing enterprise*. Keynote address, Enterprising Britain Conference. Retrieved from http://www.hm-treasury.gov.uk/ent_entconf_gates.htm

Gustafsson, L-K., & Stenberg, M. (2017). Crucial contextual attributes of nursing leadership towards a care ethics. *Nursing Ethics, 24*(4), 419–429. doi:10.1177/0969733015614879

Hawke, R. J. L. (1979). *The resolution of conflict* (1979 Boyer Lectures). Sydney: Australian Broadcasting Commission.

Institute of the Sisters of Mercy, Australia. (2007). Retrieved from http://www.mercy.org.au

Keating, P., & National Press Club (Australia). (1990). *Paul Keating address at the National Press Club, Canberra, May 9, 1990* [sound recording].

Light, S. (2009). *War diary: Matron-in-chief, British Expeditionary Force, France and Flanders*. Retrieved from http://www.scarletfinders.co.uk/110.html

McCarthy, P. M. (1986). McCarthy, Dame Emma Maud (1859–1949). *Australian dictionary of biography online edition*. Retrieved from http://www.adb.online.anu.edu.au/biogs/A100210b.htm

Piggott, J. (1990). Queen Alexandra's Royal Army Nursing Corps. In B. Horrocks (Ed.), *Famous regiments*. London, UK: Leo Cooper Ltd.

Shaw, S. (2007). *International Council of Nurses: Nursing leadership*. Oxford, UK: Blackwell Publishing.

Shields, L. (1999). Celebrating nursing achievement: Sister Mary Dorothea Sheehan RSM 1916–1999. *Neonatal, Pediatric and Child Health Nursing, 2*(4), 5–7.

Shun, K. (1995). Lao-Tzu. In T. Hondereich (Ed.), *The Oxford companion to philosophy*. Oxford, UK: Oxford University Press.

Solbakken, R., Bergdahl, E., Rudolfsson, G., & Bondas, T. (2018). International nursing: Caring in nursing leadership: A meta-ethnography from the nurse leader's perspective. *Nursing Administration Quarterly, 42*(4), E1–E19. doi:10.1097/NAQ.0000000000000314

Stanley, D., & Stanley, K. (2018). Clinical leadership and nursing explored: A literature search. *Journal of Clinical Nursing, 27*(9–1), 1730–1743. doi:10.1111/jocn.14145

Taplin, O. (1986). Homer. In J. Boardman, J. Griffin, & O. Murray (Eds.), *The Oxford history of the classical world*. Oxford, UK: Oxford University Press.

The London Hospital. (1894). Emma Maud McCarthy, September 1891–October 1894. In *London Hospital Probationer Register*. Royal London Hospital Archives, Reference LH/N/1/4.

University of Hull. (2018) Professor Roger Watson. Retrieved from http://www. hull.ac.uk/Faculties/staff-profiles/Professor-Roger-Watson.aspx

Vasak, L. (2010). Just doing my job, says VC winner Mark Donaldson. *The Australian*, January 4, 2010. Retrieved from http://www.theaustralian.com.au/news/nation/just-doing-my-job-says-vc-winner-mark-donaldson/story-e6frg6nf-1225815745839

Watson, R. (2008). Editorial: Will there ever be a Nobel Prize in nursing? *Journal of Clinical Nursing, 17*(5), 565–566. doi:10.1111/j.1365-2702.2007.02245.x

# Using Resilience as a Tool for Systemic Change

Margaret McAllister and Donna Lee Brien

## INTRODUCTION

"Wicked" problems occur not just for patients in healthcare services, as can be seen in Chapter 1, Resilience in Nursing, but also for nurses in attempting to change and improve their own professional culture. Nursing's advancement and professionalization has been hampered by internal and external tensions, including professional disunity, public misunderstanding and devaluation, and lack of political will and support to improve conditions (Thorne, 2015). This situation leads to further problems, such as stress, conflict, and burnout, and defensive coping mechanisms that can metamorphose into uncaring behaviors toward patients. It is these "wicked" problems of stress, burnout, and conflict that we focus on in this chapter.

In nursing, the constant pressure of healthcare work and the multiple demands of the many people involved (as can be seen in Chapter 5, Practicing Ethical Decision-Making) can be wearing and frustrating for nurses. It is not always possible to meet every person's needs. Furthermore, sometimes the needs of nurses are overlooked due to the unrelenting needs of suffering patients and busy clinicians.

Yet self-care is vital for nurses if they are to be able to go on caring for others, and to have the energy to solve entrenched problems. This is why the idea that resilience is equivalent to simply rolling with the punches is inadequate and insufficient. Nurses who simply roll with the punches are effectively allowing the status quo to go on.

A more fitting concept of resilience is the strength that comes from both individual *and* collective responses, activating psychological as well as social problem-solving. This definition offers a more comprehensive, and targeted, approach to overcoming these "wicked" nursing problems. Patients with complex needs (as was seen in Chapter 7, Building Resilience in Challenging Healthcare Situations, and Chapter 8, Developing Resilience in Individuals, Services, and Systems), whose problems may be familial, intergenerational, cultural, or connected to systemic unresolved injustice, are not helped by nurses who simply care for those patients' immediate, biological needs. A wider vision, informed by history, the social determinants of health, equity, and ethics are needed.

A story about one nurse's reaction to nursing stress follows.

### The Stafford Hospital Saga

In 2002, when Helené Donnelly joined the staff of the accident and emergency department (A&E) of Stafford Hospital as a newly registered nurse, she had two aspirations: first, to deliver excellent care to others, and, second, to create a successful nursing career for herself. Unfortunately, it did not take her long to realize that this hospital had a very different culture to the one she trained within. Here, economic savings were a much higher priority and quality control mechanisms and local leadership were poor. Despite strict policies to ensure patients waited no longer than 4 hours in the emergency department, staffing levels were low, their skill mixes uneven, and access to training and development minimal. Junior staff were terrified by the amounts and level of work expected of them but were too frightened to speak up because they would be openly ridiculed by the two sisters in charge. Nursing staff lacked both support and any adequate supervision, had to work with defective equipment, and could not possibly meet the patient-throughput targets expected. Rather than acknowledge that these targets could not be reached, staff were coerced by managers into fudging the data and falsifying the length of time that patients waited.

Over the next few years, numerous near-misses and errors occurred that Helené duly reported by completing healthcare incident reports. She also channeled her energy into qualifying as a nurse practitioner. But her reports and complaints fell on deaf ears. Helené later reflected that in the space of 6 years, she had logged 100 incident reports—every one of them unanswered and every one of them, presumably, unaddressed. By that time, Helené realized that, in her hospital, rather than a culture of support and learning, bullying and intimidation had been longstanding, and the mistakes and neglect were becoming difficult to ignore. The medical doctors became more sympathetic to the concerns, and the groundswell of complainants were at last becoming difficult to ignore.

An internal review was undertaken and the two charge nurses were suspended, pending evidence review. In this tense climate, threats were made on Helené's life. Rather than give in, however, Helené had her husband or parents escort her to and from the entrance to the hospital each shift for protection and kept working.

Sadly, however, the internal review and its report came to nothing. Anonymous complainants meant that evidence could not be followed up. Junior doctors were advised by senior medical staff to stay out of the issue or risk damaging their careers. All retracted their statements. Essentially, staff at all levels became passive bystanders to a situation that was later described as "a litany of failure, neglect, insensitivity and ineptitude" (Campbell, 2010). To make matters worse, the offending nursing leaders were soon reinstated in their positions, punished with nothing more than private admonishment. The practice of falsifying records resumed, albeit more surreptitiously. Disillusioned and exhausted, Helené felt she had no other choice but to resign. She left the hospital in July 2008.

The stress, conflict, and burnout in this story are palpable. Helené and her few supporters faced barrier after barrier as they attempted to implement professional care. Rather than supervisors and policies facilitating their work, they were obstructive. Many staff felt pressured into silence, afraid to object to impractical policies and faulty equipment. Like others in similar situations, they likely feared confrontation, ridicule, and recrimination. The contract and junior staff were afraid of losing their jobs and may have been thinking that argument would only further ignite hostility and make their work even more unbearable. In refusing to acquiesce to a cynical and toxic culture, Helené took the only route possible—to defend herself and continue to make formal complaints. When stress such as this is unrelenting, exhaustion (or burnout) is the result (Cherniss, 2016). Some staff try to cope by disengaging, turning a blind eye, displacing their stress (often by blaming others), or using distancing strategies, such as operating, as it is said, "on automatic pilot." This latter phenomenon is described by social analysts as *presenteeism* (Becher & Dollard, 2016) and is linked to reduced performance and unhappiness. These defensive coping practices may relieve stress in the short term, but the root cause of the stress is unaddressed and, inevitably, the stress recurs, perhaps further depleting optimism and purpose.

> *Unconscious patterns of behavior are those that create the greatest damage. A key strategy to empower your practice is to be a mindful practitioner—conscious of your feelings, conscious of your actions.*

Helené refused all of these compromised responses and had implemented most of the textbook strategies to deal with stress and conflict—finding a productive outlet, marshaling her social resources, and staying true to her values and ideals (Cherniss, 2016)—but the situation did not only not resolve. It got worse. Rightly, she came to believe that resolution was not possible on her own.

## WAYS TO RESIST STRESS AND BURNOUT

Drawing on this story as an example, it is clear that the hospital culture was contributing to stress, rather than alleviating it. Colleagues were defensive and closed to each other rather than open and supportive. Very little compassion was flowing from nurses either to themselves or others. Peers were unsupportive and there was no evidence that the problem at hand was being dealt with in a collective or productive way.

### Create Healthy Environments

Nurses are routinely subject to significant amounts of stress from sources emanating from the suffering of others, and directed at them through bullying, intimidation, and violence (Marshall, Craig, & Meyer, 2017).

This creates a psychologically unsafe work environment. Recent research by Safe Work Australia (Becher & Dollard, 2016) reported that productivity has been declining in the past decade because most Australian workers believe their workplace is not psychologically safe. Not addressing psychosocial issues places a burden on society and organizations. The cost of untreated psychological health problems on Australian organizations is approximately $10.9 billion per year, through absenteeism, presenteeism, and workers' compensation.

Psychosocial safety climate (PSC) is a recently identified aspect of organizational climate. PSC supports psychological health through policies and practices within an organization that arise from feedback from listening to workers' concerns and prioritizing and protecting their mental health over production demands.

*Too many nurses leave the profession early in their career—hurt by adverse events, alienated by an impersonal or uncaring workplace. You can make a difference to this culture, by being positive, surrounding yourself with people who care about you, and enacting small changes that build a supportive culture.*

It is disturbing that nurses have a higher rate of injury compensation than any other professional or paraprofessional group in healthcare (Peterson, 2007), and appear to suffer the most burnout. Interestingly, however, this stress is rarely related to patient problems (Regan, Howard, & Oyebode, 2009).

While sources of stress are sometimes emanating from external pressures such as the burden of care and a high level of anxiety in others, some other difficulties that nurses face are a result of their own actions and attitudes; that is, they are self-made or at least unmanaged, which leads to another strategy—the need for self-care.

## Practice Good Self-Care

Although caring is central to nursing practice, many nurses neglect self-care (Mills, Wand, & Fraser, 2015) and, indeed, self-sacrifice is viewed as noble (Rowe & Kidd, 2009). But as was outlined in Chapter 11,

Maintaining Your Resilience, efforts to maintain and express positive emotions and to practice and model well-being behaviors may have a positive impact on the individual nurse and the nursing team. Self-care thus transforms from an individualistic to cultural practice.

Self-care, which is the self-initiated behaviors that are consciously applied to promote holistic health and well-being (Mills et al., 2018), is also not limited to coping with stress. Self-care is physical, psychological, social, and spiritual. Self-care prevents ill-health, and enhances the capacity to bounce back from pressures, and, if trauma or ill-health does arrive, can facilitate a faster return to health (Figure 13.1). Thus, it is a practice that is useful in the everyday as well as when extraordinary events occur.

Self-care may include physical actions such as including recommended levels of exercise, nutrition, hydration, and sleep in daily activities. Psychological actions include meditation and positive-self-talk. Spiritual actions include efforts to find meaning and purpose in life, and to contemplate how one's life fits within a grander or larger schema. Self-care may also include the maintenance of work–life harmony. This is the idea that work and personal life are two aspects that may not always exist in equal balance all of the time, but they can be harmonious. This may mean *focusing more* on work sometimes in order to consciously give life meaning, and provide a sense of achievement and worth, and at other times in life it may be important to focus more on family. In building this harmony it is vital for nurses to actively and intentionally build a work–life where they are working with people who understand, support, like, and respect them *and* vice versa. All of these actions help to cultivate a working life that is productive, supportive, *and* enjoyable (Hill & Carroll, 2014).

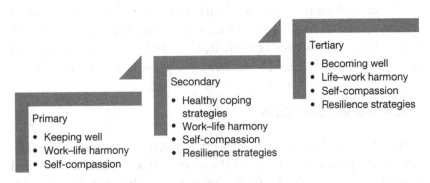

**Figure 13.1** Self-care strategies across the health spectrum.

Self-care also involves self-compassion. Where compassion is a universal feeling for, and witnessing of, the suffering of others (Larkin, 2016), self-compassion is compassion directed inwardly using kindness, patience, and understanding (Germer, 2009). It provides an important counter-balance to the tendency for self-criticism and negative judgment when expectations are not met. Self-compassion allows one to see that experiences such as disappointment, failure, or errors are part of the common human experience. Finally, self-compassion offers a way to be mindful and aware of painful thoughts and feelings, without overidentifying or succumbing to them (Neff & Dahm, 2015).

The practice of gratitude is another positive emotion that has flow-on physical benefits. Numerous studies have shown that cultivating gratitude improves relaxation, sleep, and optimism (Jackowska, Brown, Ronaldson, & Steptoe, 2015; Mills et al., 2015), and the more that positive emotions are developed, the greater the mind's flexibility and openness to change (Fredrickson, 2001). Being open to change and new things allows the possibility for widening one's repertoire of sources of support (Fredrickson, 2008).

## Build Support Networks

Stress continues to flow when it is simply repressed or ignored. When stress is projected or displaced onto other targets, such as onto nursing colleagues and assistants, stress becomes cyclical and is known as horizontal violence (Freire, 1972) in nursing. After experiencing this kind of working relationship regularly, many nurses may quite possibly unconsciously mirror the same coping style. Thus, this nurse unconsciously becomes the stereotype of the gruff but efficient nurse, who unintentionally intimidates or frightens students and new graduates—putting some of them off nursing for life. Such behavior also contributes considerably to burnout.

As Freire (1972) explains, horizontal violence is nonphysical intragroup conflict that is manifested in overt (clear) and covert (more hidden) behaviors of hostility. Horizontal violence is a characteristic of oppressed groups who have a sense of powerlessness and perceived inability to resolve their tension or problems directly with the oppressor.

But, of course, there are other behaviors to choose from when faced with stress, harassment, or interpersonal conflict. It is fascinating to imagine what Florence Nightingale or Mary Seacole (discussed in Chapter 2, Historical Models of Resilience) might have done when faced with the kind of system-wide dysfunction evident within Helené's story. Very likely they would have responded assertively and proactively. They would have assembled the team and reminded them of their higher duties—not just with the patients at hand, but within society to become role models of efficiency and effectiveness.

Being prosocial role models also has a positive feedback effect. The more respected a person feels, the more they may respect both themselves and their team. This respect can be further developed by nurturing relationships with colleagues. Their unconditional support provides a safe haven for letting off emotional steam. Connecting with colleagues gives individuals opportunities to relate, vent about stressful situations, and reaffirm that they are not alone in dealing with the trials and tribulations of the work environment. Just being able to talk to someone who has seen what you have seen, cared the way you have cared, or suffered the way you have suffered can ease the situation, and help you work through your stress and frustrations and let them go. Colleagues with more experience can provide guidance and insights into challenging situations and can provide a colleague to explore positive solutions with. Finding a trusted professional colleague with whom to share experiences also provides a nurturing relationship for that person as well.

## HELENÉ DONNELLY'S STORY CONTINUES

Even though Helené had given up her fight with managers and left Stafford Hospital, unknown to her, others—including family members of patients who had suffered and died in the hospital were inspired to keep protesting and to refuse inaction. In 2009, a group was established called "Cure the NHS" comprising relatives, patients, and community members (Cure the NHS, 2018). Together, they set up a campaign and used social media, media communications, and government lobbying to plead for a public inquiry. Eventually, they succeeded. The National Independent Healthcare Commission ordered a public inquiry, which gathered evidence from many sources.

With a new job and a baby on the way, Helené could have just walked away. But instead, her moral code once again was activated and she willingly approached the Commission and became a key witness during the inquiry. Her evidence was vital.

The commissioner, Robert Francis, Q.C., ultimately exposed scandalous reports of neglectful care: harassed, uncaring nursing staff who had lost the sight of their fundamental obligation to care (Wright, 2013). Nurses and healthcare assistants did not bother to help feeding patients who were unable to do so on their own, water was left out of reach while persistent requests for help were ignored. Medicines were prescribed but not given, patients were discharged without being fit to go home, while those left behind were often left unwashed and unfed. "The most basic standards of care were not observed and fundamental rights to dignity were not respected," Francis stated (2013). In all, 1,200 preventable deaths were reported to have occurred in this hospital over a 3-year period. All these deaths were due to neglect and inferior care. Helené's outrage—and all her complaints—were finally corroborated.

The public inquiry was the catalyst for significant cultural change across the NHS and, in particular, at Stafford Hospital. Structures were put into place to ensure that patients' interests were prioritized above budgets and meeting targets. Communication pathways were restructured to ensure that finance and quality assurance departments regularly interacted and that if lapses in care occurred, these would be reported and immediately dealt with.

Helené Donnelly now leads a new post at Stafford Hospital. She has been made an Ambassador for Cultural Change, where she has a clear remit to act freely and with autonomy to raise standards of professionalism across the hospital. She reports only to the board of directors, to whom she has immediate access to report any issue of concern. As a result of the situation that was uncovered at Stafford hospital, such positions have been rolled out right across the NHS. In 2014, Helene was awarded an Order of the Briitsh Empire in recognition of her work to support hospital staff and improve patient care (Gillen, 2014).

There are two additional important strategies evident within the conclusion of this story that we hope resonate and are remembered. They are that: (a) heroic action, while calling on courage and risk from passionate individuals, is a preferred action to doing nothing and allowing harm to occur within healthcare; and (b) collective action is a strategic resilience practice that prompts change through pressure and persistence and protects the rights of individual workers.

## Becoming a Hero Rather Than a Bystander

Sources of stress are never-ending in nursing. The impact of that stress on nursing staff requires proactive leadership in order to prevent and manage it. As Helené Donnelly's story shows, this involves courage, risk taking, and both protective and restorative interventions. Such actions are characteristics of heroism (Allison, Goethals, & Kramer, 2016). In contemporary culture, heroes are often thought of as extraordinary individuals who overcome injustice or apathy by marshaling their courage and outrage to act strategically and defensively to save another person's life, regardless of the peril they put themselves in.

Nurses need to act courageously in the workplace and refuse to be bystanders and watch unfair or distressing things happen to vulnerable people. At times this might be uncomfortable, but it is not reasonable or feasible to expect nurses to always sacrifice their own well-being for others. Rather than thinking about a hero performing extraordinary actions—such as rerouting a train from going over a cliff or disarming a gang of terrorists—nurses can be inspired to enact more effectively in leadership roles if they have a greater understanding of the role of heroic action in their everyday working lives. If the system is to be changed, learning how and when to become—or contribute to—heroic leadership is vital. Kinsella, Richie, and Igou (2015) found that the central features that heroes share are moral integrity, bravery, and self-sacrifice.

## Take Collective Action

As has been discussed in this book, sometimes problems arise within healthcare that have more to do with the structural inequities and erosion of ethics than any individual issue or specific action. To act alone in the face of such problems can not only be dangerous personally and professionally, it can be ineffective, because a solitary voice is easy to ignore.

Professional organizations allow individual workers the protection afforded by the group's structure, and the support of the group of members. Being a member of nursing organizations gives an individual nurse a group to air complaints to, find validation or correction of one's perceptions and, importantly, an avenue to issues with employers and policy makers without the risk of personal recriminations.

In Australia, the Australian College of Nursing, and in North America, the American Nurses Association, are the peak professional bodies representing nurses. These bodies work to improve the education and professional status of nurses. They are also trade unions that lobby for, and protect, workers' (in this case, nurses') rights and industrial conditions. While in this book we have focused on the stressors and issues with nursing in performing these tasks and roles, professional nursing organizations have triggered and sustained changes that have significantly advanced and enhanced the status of nursing. For example, using the power of a collective voice and strategically targeting members of relevant governments, in many countries nursing organizations have successfully obtained university education for nurses. The benefit of this training cannot be underestimated for nurses and nursing. This has ensured equal access to learning that other health colleagues had taken for granted for many years, and has also meant that nursing can no longer be considered *a calling* that needed little recompense—a sexist and anachronistic position (Raatikainen, 1997). Now, nurses expect and are given equal access to quality tertiary-level teaching and learning, and employers must provide wages and conditions such as penalty rates for shift work, incremental wage raises for experience and increased responsibilities, and superannuation. They must also ensure safe working conditions and follow other professional standards.

Over the years, various industrial organizations and their members have fought hard to not only maintain, but also improve, working conditions for nurses. An example is the 2015 Queensland Campaign in Australia—*Ratios Save Lives*—that drew on studies that showed that qualified nurses, working with a minimum nurse-to-patient ratio, led to lower patient mortality and morbidity rates than wards staffed by unqualified nurses with no limits to the numbers of patients being cared for (Aiken et al., 2014). The campaign gained support from all sides of politics in the lead up to an election and set a benchmark for a roll-out presently underway across the whole of Australia (Queensland Nurses and Midwives' Union, 2018).

Although the sources of stress and adversity for nurses will continue, being part of a collective offers a source of resilience because it amplifies and strengthens nurses' voices and can also provide an antidote to burnout. Being a member of a professional organization also gives individuals access to change strategies, as well as influence and decision-making powers that can be utilized when irrational or unfair practices at work become overwhelming or unsolvable at the site-specific or local level.

A number of documentary films chronicle both the struggles and triumphs of collective action in nursing. These are not only fascinating to watch and learn about their actions but also about the strategies that nurses have used to push back against unfairness or poor conditions. *Power of the Nurses* (Thieme, 2010) is, for instance, a documentary about the first strike by the Maine State Nursing Association when, in 2010, nurses in this association went on strike about unsafe staffing practices including patient-to-nurse ratios that were too high. Apart from its content, the title of this film is suggestive, too, relating to both common sense and recent research that backs up the assertion that power in nursing has a "determining effect on the achievement of professional goals" (Sepasi, Borhani, & Abbaszadeh, 2017, p. 4853). This research found that the ability to have, and utilize, power is "essential for promoting the roles of nurses, improving their professional image and the consistent improvement of healthcare systems" (p. 4853). Such power can moreover only be gained through a focus on the "human, ethical, professional, individual and organizational capacities" of nurses (p. 4858).

## CONCLUSION

A range of resilience strategies are illustrated in the workplace stories throughout this book. One of the significant benefits of storytelling for learning is that it is far easier to remember a well-told story than it is to remember lists or facts or figures. At some time in every reader's career, it will be useful to recall and apply these strategies, which will be important for their well-being.

*Stories can embody lessons and, if they are rich, you will remember them for life. To help future nursing students and colleagues, share the stories that motivated and inspired you.*

Without the ethical reasoning skills that were discussed in Chapter 5, Practicing Ethical Decision-Making, nurses are vulnerable to feeling the tension of dilemmas and simply do not know how best to respond.

As explained in Chapter 6, Appraising and Moderating Stressful Situations, everyone has different reactive styles to events, and each person can—in his or her own work role—challenge and replace unhelpful or ineffective cognitions. Not only can a person's own cognitive distortions be challenged and replaced, we can all also positively influence others' beliefs. When biases and expectations are suspended and other people are listened closely to, they will feel that their concerns have been heard. Additionally, this means that the listener is not simply confirming his or her own preconceived judgments and expectations, but is taking on board others' points of view. This is a useful chapter to refer to in situations whenever a reader finds himself or herself attributing reasons for other peoples' disappointing or upsetting behavior to a single source. Nurses work in very busy environments, with many colleagues, each with a pressing job to do. When conflict or tension occurs, rather than take a blaming approach to the individual, it is much more productive to try to reflect on possible sources of rising tension. It is also important to appreciate that most of the time in healthcare, good people are trying their best to complete a very difficult job.

The stories in Chapter 9, Activating Resilience Under Stress, explain that nurses work in an environment that is often highly emotionally charged. This is, in part, due to how the nursing role involves the intertwining of two selves—a professional and a personal self. Nurses do not leave their own personality or their own values at home when they start the working day, nor do their team mates who work with them. One reason that workplace tension develops is because team members come to the work with differing priorities, and various personal situations, and not all of these priorities are familiar to other team members.

It is important to remember that nurses do not have to struggle alone to find meaning in these challenges. Professional networks can provide a safe venue for discussing interpersonal problems productively. Collaborative action is much more effective than working alone on an entrenched problem as, for instance, in the case of a nurse experiencing unfairness. Once this is revealed within that nurse's group, the members can name the problem, validate their feelings, and collaborate on rectifying the situation.

And when the busy day is over nurses need to relax, unwind, and get on with living the other parts of their lives that they need to be fulfilled, happy, connected, and valued human beings. This is where all the advice about happy, healthy work–life harmony—including about diet, exercise, relaxation, hobbies, and relationships—is useful to consider and follow whichever parts of this advice are appropriate.

It is important to never forget, however, that nursing, like all of the health professions, is difficult work. There will be times when even the best relaxation measures and strategies will not help someone sleep at night. There is grief and heartache ahead for all nurses because nursing is about caring for people when they are at their most vulnerable. Nurses work at the scene of the diagnosis, inciden,t and the accident. They are there through the night when reality hits the client facing an uncertain or frightening prognosis. They are also standing at the door when clients are discharged, only to greet another client in need, in pain, in another healthcare crisis. Some, no matter what care they receive, will not respond to this care and will die. Many nurses thrive in this dynamic environment, but sometimes even the most experienced can be caught by surprise, and wounded by events to which they thought themselves immune. Many stories like that of Helené Donnelly's may become lifelong memories. If meaning is searched for, and found, in these stories, they will provide powerful and positive lessons about the standards a nurse refuses to walk past; the patient whom a nurse couldn't save, but who touched a chord deep within when he thanked the nurse for being gentle; the family member who displayed selflessness when their second child was diagnosed with a life-threatening disease; the clinician who uttered just a simple word or two to his colleague, somehow making everything seem much more manageable and okay.

This blend of assertion and compassion are characteristic traits of good leaders and of everyday acts of heroism (Keczer, File, Orosz, & Zimbardo, 2016). The development of positive leadership strategies is yet another resilience strategy that helps to empower nursing practice. As discussed in Chapter 10, Fostering Resilience in Others, leadership is not restricted to those who hold positions of legitimate authority. Nurses regularly work in teams, thus learning to be a loyal and supportive follower will be a vital resilience skill. In Chapter 12, Leading a Resilient Nursing Workforce, it was revealed that leaders who hold legitimate authority must also be able to be one of the people. Sister Dorothea was just as ready to provide cups of tea to tired nurses as she was to fight robustly for a cause in high level management meetings. It is instructive to also recall Maria Stromberger, the nurse who demonstrated incredible courage during the Second World War. Leadership is a quality available to all. As a reader and a nurse, now that you have finished this book, you have the knowledge and strategies to become a resilient, empowered nurse. We hope that you will choose to call to mind effective leaders, integrate their qualities into your own practice, and ultimately become the kind of nurse who will support, listen, understand and inspire others. In the not-too-distant future, you may be the team leader who greets new graduates on their very first day. By enjoying the challenge of helping them grow, you will embody the image of the empowered nurse that was the vision and hope behind this book. We wish you the very best in your nursing career—as an empowered individual, it is yours to create!

## LEARNING ACTIVITIES

1. In this chapter, a case study is examined of the impact a dysfunctional hospital culture has on staff—the Staffordshire Hospital. Of course, patients are the primary people harmed by poor standards of care. View the related documentary and discuss the way this dysfunction unfolded, and its impact: www .youtube.com/watch?v=iHXOFS9ec2Q
2. Imagine you were a group of nurses, working in this context. Working in small groups, draw on the cognitive and psychosocial skills suggested in this chapter to plan an approach to change that operates at three levels: patient, nurse, and system.
3. Holism is a philosophy that fits the values and aspirations of nursing. However, the pathogenic or deficit model—has a dominant influence in hospital and health service structures and processes. Compare and contrast the values, aims, strategies and outcomes of both.
4. A major responsibility for nurses is to work collaboratively with vulnerable groups. But when nurses lack confidence to advocate for fairness and justice, their disempowerment flows on to patients. Nonassertive nurses may engage in bystander apathy, which allows inequity to continue. Discuss how the concept of the alternative to bystander apathy—heroic action— can be put into place in the every-day work of nurses.

# REFERENCES

Aiken, L. H., Sloane, D. M., Bruyneel, L., Van den Heede, K., Griffiths, P., Busse, R., ... McHugh, M. (2014). Nurse staffing and education and hospital mortality in nine European countries: A retrospective observational study. *The Lancet, 383*(9931), 1824–1830. doi:10.1016/S0140-6736(13)62631-8

Allison, S. T., Goethals, G. R., & Kramer, R. M. (2016). Setting the scene: The rise and coalescence of heroism science. In S. T. Allison & R. M. Kramer (Eds.), *Handbook of heroism and heroic leadership* (pp. 1–17). New York, NY: Routledge.

Becher, H., & Dollard, M. (2016). Psychosocial safety climate and better productivity in Australian workplaces: Costs, productivity, presenteeism, absenteeism. *Safe Work Australia*. Retrieved from https://www.safeworkaustralia.gov.au

Campbell, D. (2010, February 25). NHS trust's litany of failure, neglect, insensitivity and ineptitude. *The Guardian*. Retrieved from https://www.theguardian.com/society/2010/feb/25/mid-staffordshire-nhs-trust

Cherniss, C. (2016). *Beyond burnout: Helping teachers, nurses, therapists and lawyers recover from stress and disillusionment*. London, UK: Routledge.

Cure the NHS. (2018). *Cure the NHS: Campaigning for better NHS Care*. Retrieved from http://www.curethenhs.co.uk/cure-the-nhs-campaign

Francis, R. (2013). *Report of the Mid Staffordshire NHS Foundation Trust public inquiry: Executive summary* (Vol. 947). London, UK: The Stationery Office.

Fredrickson, B. (2001). The role of positive emotions in positive psychology: The broaden and build theory of positive emotions. *American Psychologist, 56*(3), 218–226. doi:10.1037/0003-066X.56.3.218

Fredrickson, B. (2008). Promoting positive affect. In M. Eid & R. Larsen (Eds.), *The science of subjective well-being* (pp. 449–468). New York, NY: Guilford Press.

Freire, P. (1972). *Pedagogy of the oppressed*. Harmondsworth, UK: Penguin.

Germer, C. (2009). *The mindful path to self-compassion*. New York, NY: Guilford Press.

Gillen, S. (2014). A year of honours, remembrance and a historic strike over pay. *Nursing Standard, 29*(16), 14. doi:10.7748/ns.29.16.14.s19

Hill, E. J., & Carroll, S. J. (2014). Work-life harmony. In A. Michalos (Ed.), *Encyclopedia of quality of life and well-being research* (pp. 7237–7238). Netherlands: Springer.

Jackowska, M., Brown, J., Ronaldson, A., & Steptoe, A. (2015). The impact of a brief gratitude intervention on subjective well-being, biology and sleep. *Journal of Health Psychology, 21*(10), 2207–2217. doi:10.1177/1359105315572455

Keczer, Z., File, B., Orosz, G., & Zimbardo, P. G. (2016). Social representations of hero and everyday hero: A network study from representative samples. *PloS One, 11*(8), e0159354. doi:10.1371/journal.pone.0159354

Kinsella, E. L., Ritchie, T. D., & Igou, E. R. (2015). Zeroing in on heroes: A prototype analysis of hero features. *Journal of Personality and Social Psychology, 108*(1), 114. doi:10.1037/a0038463

Larkin, P. (2016). *Compassion: The essence of palliative and end-of-life-care*. Oxford, UK: Oxford University Press.

Marshall, B., Craig, A., & Meyer, A. (2017). Registered nurses' attitudes towards, and experiences of, aggression and violence in the acute hospital setting. *Kai Tiaki Nursing Research, 8*(1), 31.

Mills, P., Redwine, L., Wilson, K., Pung, M., Chinh, K., Greenberg, B., & Chopra, D. (2015). The role of gratitude in spiritual well-being in asymptomatic heart failure patients. *Spirituality in Clinical Practice, 2*(1), 5–17. doi:10.1037/scp0000050

Mills, J., Wand, T., & Fraser, J. (2018). Examining self-care, self-compassion, and compassion for others: A cross-sectional survey of palliative care nurses and doctors. *International Journal of Palliative Nursing, 24*(1), 4–11. doi:10.12968/ijpn.2018.24.1.4

Neff, K., & Dahm, K. (2015). Self-compassion: What it is, what it does, and how it relates to mindfulness. In B. Ostafin, M. Robinson, & B. Meier (Eds.), *Mindfulness and self-regulation* (pp. 121–137). New York, NY: Springer.

Peterson, C. L. (2007). Work-related stress in Australia. In C. Uyeda (Ed.), *Australian master OHS and environment guide* (2nd ed., pp. 319–335). Sydney, Australia: CCH Publishers.

Queensland Nurses and Midwives' Union. (2018). *Ratios save lives.* Retrieved from https://www.qnmu.org.au/QNMU/Campaigns/Ratios_Save_Lives/QNMU/PUBLIC/CAMPAIGNS/Ratios_Save_Lives_C1.aspx

Raatikainen, R. (1997). Nursing care as a calling. *Journal of Advanced Nursing, 25*(6), 1111–1115. doi:10.1046/j.1365-2648.1997.19970251111.x

Regan, A., Howard, R. A., & Oyebode, J. R. (2009). Emotional exhaustion and defense mechanisms in intensive therapy unit nurses. *The Journal of Nervous and Mental Disease, 197*(5), 330–336. doi:10.1097/NMD.0b013e3181a20807

Rowe, L., & Kidd, M. (2009). *First do no harm: Being a resilient doctor in the 21st century.* Maidenhead, UK: McGraw-Hill.

Sepasi, R. R., Borhani, F., & Abbaszadeh, A. (2017). Nurses' perception of the strategies to gaining professional power: A qualitative study. *Electronic Physician, 9*(7), 4853–4861. doi:10.19082/4853

Thieme, E. (2010). *Power of the nurses.* Retrieved from https://www.youtube.com/watch?v=W6iyLzSL6Bc

Thorne, S. (2015). Does nursing represent a unique angle of vision? If so, what is it? *Nursing Inquiry, 22*(4), 283–284. doi:10.1111/nin.12128

Wright, O. (2013, February 6). The Frances Report: Key findings. *The Independent.* Retrieved from https://www.independent.co.uk/life-style/health-and-families/health-news/the-francis-report-key-findings-8484071.html

# Index